LIVING WITH ASPERGER SYNDROME

JOAN GOMEZ is Honorary Consulting Psychiatrist to the Chelsea and Westminster Hospital and an established Sheldon author. Previous books include *Coping with Thyroid Problems* (1994), *Living with Diabetes* (1995) and *Coping with Incontinence* (2003). She lives in Farnham, Surrey.

Overcoming Common Problems Series

Selected titles

A full list of titles is available from Sheldon Press,
36 Causton Street, London SW1P 4ST and on our website at
www.sheldonpress.co.uk

Overcoming Common Problems

Living with Asperger Syndrome

Joan Gomez

sheldon **PRESS**

First published in Great Britain in 2005

Sheldon Press
36 Causton Street
London SW1P 4ST

British Library Cataloguing-in-Publication Data

A catalogue record for this book is available from the British Library

ISBN 0–85969–935–8

1 3 5 7 9 10 8 6 4 2

Typeset by Deltatype Limited, Birkenhead, Merseyside
Printed in Great Britain by
Ashford Colour Press

Contents

Abbreviations

ABA	Applied Behavioural Analysis
AD	Attention Deficit
ADD	Attention Deficit Disorder
A i A	Allergy induced Autism
AIT	Auditory Integration Training
AS	Asperger Syndrome
ASD	Autistic Spectrum Disorder
BAP	Broader Autistic Phenotype
CAPD	Central Auditory Processing Disorder
CBT	Cognitive Behaviour Therapy
CDD	Childhood Disintegrative Disorder
HD	Hyperactivity Disorder
OASIS	Online Asperger Syndrome Information and Support
OCD	Obsessive Compulsive Disorder
ODD	Oppositional Defiant Disorder
PDD	Pervasive Developmental Disorder
SEN	Special Educational Needs
SID	Sensory Integration Disorder
SIT	Sensory Integration Training

Introduction

Ten years ago only a handful of experts in child psychiatry had even heard of Asperger Syndrome (abbreviated to AS). Today, though, the term is on everyone's lips and appears in a wide range of journals, from specialist medical and serious scientific publications to popular women's magazines. In 2003, Mark Haddon's entertaining novel, *The Curious Incident of the Dog in the Night-time*, written in 'Aspergerese', was shortlisted for the Booker Prize, then won the Whitbread Award in 2004. In the same year, Stephen Poliakoff's play received the ultimate accolade of a showing on BBC 2. The hero was Prince John, the youngest child of George V, kept under wraps all his life because of his epilepsy and what we would today consider to be AS.

What is Asperger Syndrome (AS)?

The condition arises from a quirk in the development of the brain and nervous system, and results in lifelong problems in communication with others, especially in social situations, and in forming relationships. Youngsters with AS are fascinated by particular objects, even their own fingers. Both in childhood and as adults, they harbour an intense interest in subjects that are usually too complex or too academic to appeal to ordinary, normal people – or, to use the term employed throughout this book, *neurotypicals*. Albert Einstein and Isaac Newton, both with retrospective diagnoses of AS, show this single-minded obsession with particular subjects – in their cases, gravity, matter and space.

High intelligence shines out from those with AS more often than in the general population, but it is counterbalanced by a group who have learning difficulties. Among brilliant people today who show features of the syndrome are Bill Gates, the boss of Microsoft, and Dr Temple Grandin, a woman who has done much pioneering research into AS.

Pervasive Developmental Disorders (PDD) encompass a group of around half a dozen developmental abnormalities affecting the brain and nervous system. AS is a very special member of a family of related symptoms known as *Autistic Spectrum Disorder* (*ASD*), which is used as a general term for *autism*. ASD in turn comes under the umbrella label of PDD.

What is the difference between ASD and AS?

ASD is an expansion of the word 'autism', with the phrase being an umbrella term for autism in general. This is characterized by symptoms that appear before the age of three, and usually by 30 months. Typically, the baby, usually a boy, is particularly 'good' and quiet. He does not respond to cuddles, smiles or being spoken to, and seems not to differentiate between his mother and a stranger. He is slow in learning to talk and seems to be more interested in things than in people. General problems with eating, sleeping and temper tantrums may crop up, and are often more intense than in neurotypical children.

Asperger Syndrome (AS) is a specific type of ASD. It shows some similarities to autism, but manifests itself later, sometimes not appearing fully until puberty – or it may not be recognized at all until then. There is usually little or no delay in talking, but a child with AS is poor in the use of body language, eye contact and facial expression. He seems to prefer his own company to joining in and playing with other children. Other oddities are an inflexible insistence on certain routines and an overwhelming desire for sameness in everything. The AS triad of impairments affects social behaviour, communication and imagination.

Behind every diagnosis of AS lies a puzzling story of negative tests and positive symptoms, and a family history of unusual personalities, especially in fathers, brothers and sisters. It can be a privilege and a pleasure to have an AS child to care for and help in simple physical ways, and to protect in a world that does not understand him, and vice versa. Such a child is likely to be bright, but uses his intelligence along different lines, and feels affection from a different viewpoint from a neurotypical youngster. This viewpoint can help us in our general understanding of humanity.

Children with extreme forms of PDD (for instance Rett's disorder, Childhood Disintegrative Disorder (CDD) or Fragile X syndrome), or with serious learning difficulties or severe autism, are easily recognized by teachers and classmates as being different from other children, but of course AS children are not responsible for this. Youngsters with AS have a much worse time than their peers, and are subject to bullying at school, because they are seen as psychologically normal but awkward and unfriendly.

There has been a dramatic and continuous increase in the number of recognized cases of ASD, especially since AS has aroused such intense interest. The number of children with ASD now outstrips that for Down's syndrome, and also cerebral palsy. Even the staid *British Medical Journal* currently refers to autism as an 'epidemic'. In places as far apart culturally and geographically as Saudi Arabia, Quebec and Cambridgeshire in England, the frequency of the AS variant of ASD is escalating – a further reason for its claiming so much attention.

Autism (ASD) and AS: two typical cases

Peter

Peter was a beautiful baby. After a trouble-free pregnancy, Helen, his mother, thought she was the luckiest woman in the world when she looked at his perfect, symmetrical features, with neither the wizened old-man look of some babies, nor the immature, chubby, babyish face. And he was so good too: seldom crying and taking his feeds without a murmur. Everyone said 'like father, like son', for Philip, his father, had always been the quiet, shy type. In fact, Helen looked forward to her husband coming out of his shell to play with Peter like other dads – delicious games such as 'This little piggy went to market' and 'Incy, wincy spider'.

However, this never quite happened, but Helen hugged her baby a lot to make up for it. Oddly, he felt awkward in her arms, as though he didn't fit. When she gazed lovingly at his face and tried to look into his eyes, she found they somehow always avoided hers. Her son's lack of response puzzled her and hurt her feelings, but she told herself to thank her lucky stars for the quiet nights. Peter's sight and hearing were checked and found to be normal, but he hadn't yet begun to babble or play baby games with Helen. He seemed so alone.

It was the paediatrician, several months later, who first suggested that Peter was autistic.

Rosemary

Rosemary's parents, like Peter's, were professional people. Her father was a lawyer, her mother a maths teacher. At the age of seven, Rosemary was considered 'a bad mixer'. She did not join in with the others at school and never wanted to bring any friends home to tea. Her parents were not worried, though, because as far as her schoolwork was concerned, she was well up to average – and well above it for arithmetic. English was her worst subject; she was particularly fazed by poetry 'because it says things that aren't true'.

Rosemary disliked team games, partly because she was no good at them as a result of poor co-ordination, and partly because she preferred doing things on her own. The outcome of this was that she was always the last one to be chosen when they were picking sides. This made her sad because she wanted to be popular. As she was unable to put herself in another person's place, she did not realize that she was always upsetting or annoying the other children – for instance, by saying that netball was boring, or by sulking when her team lost.

It was not as bad for Rosemary as it would have been for a boy, because she did not stand out as being very different from other girls. A couple of neurotypical girls in her class also 'hated games', so Rosemary did not seem abnormal. The snag, though, was that she did not join in girly activities either: cosy chats, giggling about boys, buying new clothes, or playing nurses.

Thinking she was helping Rosemary over a mental barrier once and for all, an enthusiastic, pro-active but inexperienced teacher tried to shame her into taking an active part and shooting at netball. Rosemary, usually so self-effacing and passive, hit the woman as hard as she could – to stop her. This ended Rosemary's stay at that school, but it did lead to the priceless gain of her having investigations that ultimately led to a diagnosis of AS – and at last gaining some sympathy for her problems and help in dealing with them.

Portrayals of autism and AS

The actor Dustin Hoffman won an Oscar for his portrayal of autism in the film *Rain Man*, and – as we have already mentioned – Mark Haddon, the writer, received the Whitbread Award for his brilliant depiction of a boy with AS. These two artists have done a great deal to help us to understand AS, in the way that they make us feel for, and almost love, their realistic fictional characters. While retaining their own neurotypical mentalities, Hoffman and Haddon have managed to enter into their subjects' minds.

There are two particular books that have been written by children who themselves have Asperger Syndrome: *Freaks, Geeks and Asperger Syndrome: A User Guide to Adolescence* by Luke Jackson, who was 13 when he wrote this, and *Asperger Syndrome, the Universe and Everything*, by Kenneth Hall, who was ten when he wrote his account. These books are wonderful achievements and give further insights into what it is like to be an 'Aspie'.

Mothers who have written about their AS children – for instance, Charlotte Moore and Brenda Boyd – give amusing, informative and sometimes daunting accounts of the impact that a child with AS has on family life. It would be marvellous if a father could be persuaded to write a book about AS, particularly as the affected children are nearly all boys, and their personalities veer towards the masculine. For instance, the specialist subjects that those with AS choose most frequently are those that neurotypical men and boys go for anyway: maths, engineering and the sciences, rather than the more imaginative subjects of history and literature. Male researchers into AS, such as Tony Attwood, and the giants of earlier days, Kanner and Asperger himself, wrote from a male standpoint, but do not have a parent–child bond of understanding.

1

The historical background

The most fundamental, fascinating mystery of all time is the working of the human mind. The Greeks, always on the ball, recognized its complexities and subtleties some 2,000 years ago. Aristotle (384–322 BC) traced a link between melancholia (depression) and creativity, which of course depends on original thought. Three hundred years later, following the same track, the Roman Seneca (4 BC–AD 65) made his famous pronouncement that genius and madness go hand in hand. These two traits, in a much milder form, could well apply today to a super-bright child with AS, but who is likely to have language difficulties.

Typically, a child with AS has severe problems in communicating with other people, even at the simplest level, so that he can appear to others to be really stupid when he is not. Also, he may have poorly developed muscular co-ordination, so that he is very clumsy. Yet he may also show remarkable dexterity and islands of intellectual brilliance in his favourite subjects. It is his own *feelings*, and especially other people's feelings, that he cannot grasp.

The painstaking piecing together of clues, plus occasional flashes of insight, has led to our present, albeit imperfect, understanding of AS and its recognition as a specific condition. This gradual process has paralleled the development of psychiatry itself, the subject concerned with unusual or faulty functioning of the brain.

When was AS first recognized?

Dementia, literally 'without mind', was an early overall term for any brain problem. Today we only apply it to the brain failure of old age, but a hundred years ago the phrase *dementia praecox* was used to describe psychological problems in younger people. *Praecox* is Latin for 'precocious'. The pejorative word 'dippy' comes from the initials DP.

It was not until the early years of the twentieth century that modern psychiatry began to emerge. This was an era of great thinkers in the field – such as Bleuler, Jaspers, Kraepelin and, later, Freud. New theories about the mind blossomed. In 1911, Eugen

1

Bleuler brought out his *Lehrbuch* (textbook) of psychiatry and by 1916 he had also coined two important new terms: *schizophrenia* and *autism*.

Schizophrenia is a major mental illness or psychosis, and the word means, literally, 'split mind'; this split is between fantasy and reality.

Autism is not an illness

Autism refers not to an illness as such, but to a psychological state of withdrawal or being considered inward-looking – almost like a large dose of shyness. Autistic thinking is a common feature of schizophrenia, and this has led to many children who showed autistic thinking and unusual behaviour, such as those with AS, being wrongly diagnosed as suffering from childhood schizophrenia. The term *schizoid* is still used to describe an inward-looking attitude or personality, but it does not mean schizophrenic – that is, having the illness of schizophrenia.

Although the concept of autism did not evolve until the twentieth century, there had long been stories about strange, wild children who had no language, and were thought to have been brought up by wolves. Romulus and Remus, the legendary twin founders of Rome, were among the first. Victor, 'the wild boy of Aveyron', was studied for a number of years by educationist Jean Marc Gaspard Itard and his pupil Edward Seguin at the turn of the nineteenth century, and in 1929 a pair of feral – that is, wild – children, Kamala and Amala, were discovered by the Reverend Singh in Midnapore in India.

Breakthroughs in our modern understanding of autism and AS

In 1926, Ewa Ssucharewa, an obscure assistant neurologist from Russia, who had the extra handicap at that time of being a woman, published a remarkable paper. It was entitled 'Schizoid Personality Disorder in Children', a description that could well have applied to autistic youngsters. Amazingly, although it foreshadowed our current intense interest in the subject, Dr Ssucharewa's study attracted little attention until it was rediscovered, only two or three years ago. At the time when the paper was written, everyone thought that autism was a form of schizophrenia and that it resulted from faulty mothering – a mistaken belief that caused immense unhappiness. However, one lone voice disagreed, that of another woman, Dr

Loretta Bender, who firmly believed that schizophrenia was due to a lag in brain development. Although autism is not regarded today as a type of schizophrenia, Dr Bender was correct in her assessment of the underlying cause of the condition. As with Dr Ssucharewa, no one at the time took much notice of a mere woman's opinion!

The big breakthrough in our modern understanding of autism and its related disorders, including AS, came in the middle of the Second World War in 1943 and 1944 via two Austrian doctors, Dr Leo Kanner, a psychiatrist, and Dr Hans Asperger, a paediatrician specializing in remedial education. Both trained in Vienna, but they never met, although Asperger did mention Kanner's paper on one occasion. They were separated by a ten-year age gap. Kanner was born in 1896, and Asperger was born in 1906 and died in 1980. Their work put both autism and AS on the map.

Kanner's cluster of symptoms

In 1943, Kanner published his landmark paper. He originally called it 'Autistic Disturbance in Affective Control'; *affective* means 'concerned with the emotions', as in the familiar term 'affection'. He later changed the title to 'Early Infantile Autism', and finally to 'Early Childhood Autism'. In his study he described, for the first time, an interesting developmental disorder in a boy called Donald. He then searched for, and found, ten more cases in children. All 11 of these children showed a similar cluster of symptoms, to which he applied the term 'autism'. They included:

- Early onset of the problem: within the first 30 months of life.
- Extreme aloneness, with an inability to form relationships ('in a world of his own').
- Delay in learning to speak, and sometimes actual mutism.
- Difficulty in using words in a meaningful fashion.
- Repetitive, stereotyped play; no imaginative 'pretend' play.
- Anxious, obsessive desire for sameness, with resistance to change.
- Islets of remarkable ability – for instance, for playing music, drawing, calculating, and especially rote memory.

Other frequent features were lack of eye contact, or such gestures as pointing; ignoring people (including parents); lack of response to smiles and cuddles; absence of facial expression; and exceptionally 'good', quiet behaviour as a baby.

Later in childhood, imaginative activities might be affected – for example, pretend play, or copying what other people do (shadowing). Other possible traits included stereotyped movements (twisting fingers, twirling body); routines and rituals; response to 'interesting' sounds, such as food frying, doors opening and shutting, but not to a human voice; *echolalia* – repeating precisely what he has just heard, even if it is long and complicated; and a good-to-excellent rote memory. A normal or especially intelligent appearance might be deceptive, and the child might have poor comprehension, despite a good vocabulary and grasp of grammar, and a tendency to use and understand words literally, with no concept of metaphor, sarcasm or jokes. Dr Kanner also noted tantrums, anxiety attacks, and over-sensitivity to sound, touch or smell.

Some very misleading misconceptions

Some of Kanner's ideas have proved to be tragic misconceptions. Most importantly, he was convinced that the cause of autism must be the fault of 'refrigerator' mothers, bringing up their children coldly, without love. You can imagine the heart-searching, self-blame and distress of an ordinary, loving mother on hearing this, wondering how on earth she could have gone so disastrously wrong. Unfortunately, this cruelly mistaken belief was generally accepted for more than twenty years, by the public at large as well as by doctors such as the late Dr Bruno Bettelheim.

Fortunately, a number of other doctors, led by Dr Bernard Rimland, strongly opposed this view. They teamed up with a group of parents, and in 1965 they founded the Autism Society of America. They refuted Kanner's suggestions about the causes of autism, and provided support for the parents. It is now accepted that autism is essentially a neurological disorder.

In 1944, Hans Asperger published his paper 'Autistic Psychopathy in Childhood'. Coincidentally, he described a syndrome closely resembling that of Kanner's study, and also by coincidence used the term 'autistic' to describe it. This has led to some confusion. Asperger's syndrome is now generally known as Asperger Syndrome, without the apostrophe and following 's', and refers to a distinct, recognizable condition. It is characterized by three types of social deficit, involving:

1 *Social interaction*: sharing conversation and activity.

2 *Social communication*: using words, gestures and expressions to convey feelings and ideas.

3 *Social imagination*: putting yourself in another person's place.

Some people regard AS as a sub-type of Kanner's autism, while others see it as a totally independent autistic disorder. Kanner's syndrome as he originally described it is often referred to as *classic autism*.

Kanner believed that all autistic children were intellectually brilliant, or at least had the potential for high intelligence if suitably encouraged. However, this was another of his damaging misconceptions. Statistical studies have shown that 66 per cent of autistic children score in the subnormal range, although some of the remaining 34 per cent do have remarkable gifts. The misleading belief that their children are near-geniuses, if only they had the key to unlock their talents, is a further cause of frustration and self-blame among those parents whose youngsters are of no more than average ability. Kanner and Asperger were both captivated and misled by these children's attractive appearance, with intelligent faces, and apparent serious-mindedness.

Most Asperger children have an IQ at least on a level with the so-called high-functioning autistics, but there is no 100 per cent certainty. Giftedness usually applies to one or two specific subjects, such as computer and other sciences, maths and music. Asperger children differ from other autistic types in having better language skills, and they can be expected to be fluent by the time they are five. Another difference between AS and autistic children is that the former often wish to make friends with their peers and other people of all ages. Unfortunately, though, they are hopeless at picking up the meaning of common metaphors, hints or jokes, or imagining how other people feel. In contrast, children with classic autism do not care about having friends. In terms of similarities, both AS and autistic children enjoy their own company.

While communicating with others means less than nothing to Kanner-type autistic children, a number of Asperger children and young adults have written books with the specific aim of explaining and sharing their thoughts and feelings. As we mentioned earlier, Kenneth Hall wrote his excellent book *Asperger Syndrome, the Universe and Everything* when he was only ten, while Luke Jackson produced his *Freaks, Geeks and Asperger Syndrome: A User Guide to Adolescence* at the age of 13.

As well as the tremendous help given to Asperger subjects by their dedicated doctors, teachers and carers – of whom the most famous was Sister Viktorine Zak at the paediatric clinic in Vienna – the parents of Asperger children have made a major contribution to our knowledge of the syndrome and the various ways of coping with it. Interestingly, in more than 40 per cent of the parents, at least one of them has had a language problem.

Hans Asperger himself was a scholar with a first-class brain and a mission to make the world a happier place for Asperger children, for whom he had a fellow feeling. Most other people regarded them as rude and unfriendly, given to rages and screaming, and extremely obstinate concerning their likes and dislikes. We now realize that this behaviour is the result of an inbuilt disability, not a deliberate desire to upset people.

In 1991, Dr Uta Frith translated Asperger's paper and presented his syndrome to the English-speaking world. This was like switching on a searchlight, and since then AS has seldom been free of media attention.

Current thinking

A group of new terms has developed around AS, reflecting modern thinking on the subject. We have already mentioned some of these phrases:

- *Pervasive Developmental Disorder (PDD)*, an umbrella concept that includes, among others, AS.
- *Autistic Spectrum Disorder (ASD)*, another inclusive term, often applied to autistic children who function well intellectually, such as those showing Asperger symptoms.
- *Broader Autistic Phenotype (BAP)*, the most recently introduced, even bigger umbrella, covering those very sketchily affected, showing only one or two of the characteristics of autism.
- *Asperger Syndrome* – official recognition in 1994! AS is described as a separate entity among the PDDs in the *Diagnostic and Statistical Manual of Mental Disorders of the American Psychiatric Association* (DSM IV). A little later, it was also included in the International Classification of Diseases (ICD 10).

Meanwhile, Asperger parents, always on the alert for ways of helping their youngsters, had cottoned on to electronic technology and the internet. E-mails keep them in touch with one another for support and to spread the word about any new developments. For example, a group of parents in south London set up a school especially for children with AS – a fascinating project.

Barbara Kirby, the mother of an eight-year-old boy diagnosed with AS, was instrumental in setting up a website specifically for those concerned with AS. It is called Online Asperger Syndrome Information and Support, known as OASIS.

So much for the history of AS – the good news is that the future looks full of promise.

Causes of AS

While the specific causes of ASD, including AS, remain a mystery, we are certain that it has a biological not a psychological basis, and strong genetic links. It is now accepted that autism is basically a neurological disorder that results from one of three causes:

1 A genetic quirk.
2 An insult or injury to the brain.
3 A brain disorder impinging on its development.

Specifically, AS has nothing to do with the dreadful old theory of cold and cruel parents, especially mothers. This has been disproved over and over again, but even today some mothers only too easily try to take the blame for their child being different from other youngsters. The theory that cold, over-intellectual treatment of the child led to ASD first arose when Professor Kanner, in 1943, noticed that the parents of autistic children tended to be highly intelligent middle-class professionals, but he was basing his judgement on the parents of only a handful of individuals – just 11 in all. With the large numbers of children included in up-to-date studies, statistics have established that children with AS come from all walks of life.

Genetic factors play a most important role as they hand down their message from generation to generation. Chromosomes 11 and 15 and the Y chromosome are thought to be implicated.

A brother or sister of a child with ASD or AS has 50 times the normal risk of having the condition, and there is a 46 per cent chance of his other first-degree relatives being affected. Fathers have the symptoms in 19 per cent of cases, though mothers in only 2 per cent.

More than a third of parents of an AS child have been diagnosed with one of the conditions *co-morbid* (in other words, associated) with the condition – for instance, depression, bipolar disorder or OCD (Obsessive Compulsive Disorder; see Chapter 7).

Statistics for twins also underline proof of a genetic factor. Concordance for autism (that is, when both twins are affected) occurs in 64 per cent of identical or monozygotic pairs, but only 10 per cent of fraternal or dizygotic pairs – a clear indication of genes at work. A seemingly unaffected twin of an identical pair has a 90–95 per cent likelihood of developing autism or a 30–40 per cent risk with a dizygotic pair.

But, while genetic inheritance is necessary, there must also be one or more biological causes – or triggers – that may damage the developing brain of the unborn child. One example is rubella (German measles), occurring when the mother is pregnant. The vulnerable areas in relation to AS are the right hemisphere, the cerebellum and, significantly, the mysterious limbic lobe that is concerned with feelings. This ties up with the problems in communication and lack of empathy in AS.

Another idea that has been thrown on the rubbish heap, but which had damaging national repercussions on the immunization pro-gramme over several years, was the theory that the MMR vaccine (measles, mumps and rubella) caused autism and Crohn's disease. It has now been established beyond all reasonable doubt that there are no such connections, and its proponents accordingly discredited. The last attempt at trotting out this outdated theory was in late 2004.

2

The numbers game: statistics

Since the identification of AS as a separate syndrome in the two main classification systems, DSM IV and ICD 10, there has been a steep rise in the number of cases recorded and also renewed interest in autism in general; this is partly a reflection of our more detailed and increasingly widespread knowledge about these conditions.

The good news is that you are not alone if you are faced with the daunting diagnosis of AS in your child. Help is at hand. The intense interest in the subject and the large numbers involved means that research into the problems is going on simultaneously and continuously, all over the world. It also means that whether you live in a bustling city or a quiet backwater, your local doctor will have read all about ASD and AS in the medical press. With so many people concerned, every new treatment, no matter how way out – for instance, swimming with dolphins, which sounds delightful – will be tried out by plenty of others and you will benefit from their experience, good or bad. You will get updates from an online or paper newsletter, the OASIS website (http://www.aspergersyndrome. org.), or your specialist.

Statistics are like good friends; you can usually trust them to tell you the truth. They will tell you what to expect – what is 'normal' or commonplace for a child, adolescent or adult diagnosed with AS. Another good thing about statistics is that it is a subject that appeals to youngsters with AS. The answers are logical and precise enough to fit into the Asperger corner in all of us.

Numbers

The numbers clearly reveal the sharp rise in our recognition of ASD over the years:

- Between 1966 and 1984 there were 0.4 cases of autism per 1,000 children in the USA.
- Between 1986 and 1997 there was an increase to 1 case in 1,000 (10 in 10,000).

Actual figures for AS
- 1966: 4–5 cases in 10,000.

- 1979: 21 cases in 10,000.
- 1989: a collection of major studies assessed that, in the Western world, between 10 and 26 children in 10,000 had AS.
- 1993: the number of cases of AS had escalated to approximately 71 in 10,000.
- 2000: a recent count puts the number of cases of AS among children in the USA and the UK at 1 in 250–500. The range is wide because the symptoms are so variable that the diagnosis is difficult to make, and there can be uncertainty and disagreement between psychiatrists – and even more so between non-specialist doctors.

Current totals for ASD, including AS

- USA: 500,000 in a population of 274 million.
- UK: 207,500 in a population of 66 million. This is, proportionately, 4 per cent more than in the USA. It has recently (2004) been hypothesized that the difference is because of a relative shortage of Vitamin D, the 'sunshine' vitamin, in the UK. In Northern Europe there is less of the sunlight necessary for the body to synthesize it.

Prevalence of autism in some northern countries

- 1991 Sweden more than 26 per 10,000.
- 1998 Sweden more than 48 per 10,000.
- 1980 Iceland more than 36 per 10,000.

The number of children with ASD in the West now exceeds that of most of the major children's disorders – for instance, Down's syndrome, childhood cancer, muscular dystrophy or cerebral palsy.

Wide differences, yet one diagnosis

What the numbers don't show is how the same diagnosis can be applied to individuals who differ widely:

Jeremy and Christopher

Jeremy, five, and Christopher, three, were brothers and both had been diagnosed with AS, but they were as different as chalk and cheese. Jeremy lived in a world of his own that he had no inclination to share. He avoided communication with others either by body language, including eye contact and facial expression, or by speaking in his characteristically literal way. The one subject that he would talk about endlessly was his favourite – timetables, whether bus, train, air or school lessons. He liked order and would arrange his toys in rows, whether soft animals or automobiles.

Christopher presented quite a different picture and was given to shouting, banging and screaming when he was thwarted. He did not play with toys, but destroyed them with concentrated energy. He would hit other people if they touched him, probably because his extreme sensitivity made any skin contact painful.

Statistics tell us nothing about feelings

The cold statistics also give no sense of the serious nature of ASD in terms of the suffering it causes both to the child and those who love him. Parents are puzzled and distressed by their child's odd and sometimes antisocial behaviour. They may be blamed either for starving him of affection, or for overindulging and spoiling him. The child with AS is aware that he is different from other people and finds them difficult to understand. Over-literal interpretation is another common cause of misunderstanding, though fortunately 'I'm dying for a cup of tea' would not mean to an Aspie that you should call an ambulance. AS is a lifelong problem, but caring, sensitive treatment can ameliorate many of the symptoms. This does not require special skills, but love in spadefuls, and patience, from a professional or parent.

Perhaps saddest of all, the child longs to be liked, but does not have the slightest social sense. Although he wants others to like him, he cannot imagine how they feel. This stops him from making friends and he may remain very much alone.

Paul
Paul wore people down with non-stop talk about his favourite subject, global warming. He fancied a girl who went to the same school, but could not think of anything appropriate to say to her, so he told her about global warming and the end of civilization. Not surprisingly, it didn't grab her.

The good news is that AS children can be taught social skills to help smooth their paths through life (see advice on helping your child to communicate in Chapter 11).

Boys and girls

As mentioned earlier, most children diagnosed as having AS are boys. The ratio is 10:1, and their interests are often so-called masculine ones: the sciences, maths, astronomy, engineering and construction and, of course, computers and the worldwide web. If you take a broader diagnosis of ASD, there is less of a male bias: 4:1 – four boys to every one girl.

More numbers

Of the 3 or 4 children in 1,000 who show the full picture of AS, only half ask for psychiatric help. In spite of the claims of latent genius in autistic and, more especially, children with AS, statistics tell us that 66 per cent of them function as mentally retarded, and 25–30 per cent have epilepsy. Epilepsy is definitely a neurological disorder, and thus it is clear evidence that AS is not just a matter of bad behaviour. It is significant that 70 per cent of parents of AS children come from professional or highly skilled backgrounds, although the majority of them have had difficulties with language development and in reading body language.

Among older children with AS, over 50 per cent are neglectful of hygiene – and have to be dragooned into cleaning their teeth and washing their hair. From about the age of ten, they are also susceptible to mild to moderate depression or irritability.

Neurobiological quirks affect 30–75 per cent of autistic children, for instance clumsiness (although some are remarkably dexterous – a common feature), tremors, odd ways of walking and standing, and hypo- or hypertonia – which means, respectively, floppy or tense muscles.

Although there are plenty of difficulties for children with AS, 60 per cent of them say that, on balance, there are more benefits than disadvantages – for instance, the ability to focus on a particular subject, or to cope with being on their own. And here is a final cheerful statistic: 80 per cent of parents come to terms with their situation and their child's AS within a year, and the children agree that it is cool to be an Aspie.

3

The family

Asperger Syndrome (AS) is a family matter, and a family usually grows out of love. It starts with two people whose lives are joined and who then have the added joy of a child. If he – or less likely, she – is one of those special children with AS, the parents are blessed indeed. This is a child who really needs what you, as a mother or father, long to give – love and understanding. You will, though, also need a generous helping of patience.

When there is a child with AS in the family everyone is affected in one way or another, especially parents, brothers and sisters, but also more distant relatives. It is a matter of the genes they share. There may be nothing about the family that stands out as different – until you take a closer look. This genetic streak will show up in subtle differences in behaviour in some family members compared with so-called normal people.

The Asperger *phenotype* is a recognizable pattern of characteristics seen only when the Asperger genes are present. It can show up in totally unrelated families, yet it is as though they all belong to one enormous, worldwide family. Such individuals often share a tendency to be quiet and reserved, and easily become anxious. Typically their thinking is logical, but literal. For example, if on a hot day you say 'I'm boiling' to a child with AS, he may point out that this is impossible, or look for the steam!

Parents

The people most affected by having a child with AS in the family are obviously the parents. At first they may feel vaguely uneasy that their little one seems different from other children of the same age, often by being extra 'good' as a baby. Sooner or later, though, the nagging suspicion that something is not quite right turns to near certainty. In many cases, around the age of three, someone – either a professional or a friend with personal experience of ASD – brings up the possibility of AS as an explanation for the child's weird or unusual behaviour.

Faced with the suggestion that their toddler has a form of autism,

13

the parents' world turns topsy-turvy. After the initial shock, they may react in a variety of ways:

1 *Denial.* They will not accept the diagnosis and argue fiercely against it. They insist that their son or daughter is perfectly normal, 'only a little shy and takes after his father'. The latter may be perfectly true – the father may have a mild case of ASD – but the child will need all the help his parents can muster and all his own courage and persistence to build a good life in spite of the inborn difficulties. No wonder some parents try to wish the AS away.

2 *Relief.* It is almost universal to feel a sense of relief when a definite diagnosis emerges. It means that your worries are being taken seriously – you were not just imagining that something was amiss.

3 *Over-protectiveness.* A wave of pity and protectiveness engulfs some parents. While it is important to look out for your child and ease his path through the inevitable social hiccups, coddling him will damage his already fragile self-confidence. It is a matter of judgement.

4 *Anger.* In this case, you look for someone to blame. The doctor? Your partner? The nursery school? It is tempting to blame someone else, but unfair criticism only causes more unhappiness as it did 160 years ago in Kanner's and Asperger's time. Parents then, especially mothers, were routinely accused of causing their child's problems by their coldness. There is not an atom of truth in this theory, but what heartache it caused.

5 *Guilt.* Innocent as they are of causing their child's AS, with the biological facts to prove it, some parents are riven by guilt and endlessly comb their memories for things they could have done differently. They need to banish these negative, illogical notions and concentrate instead on enjoying their dear, wonderful child, and instead give him the best possible start in life. A common cause of acute guilt occurs when one parent, exhausted and at the end of their tether, loses their rag. It happens to everyone occasionally under the special stress of coping day in and day out with a difficult child – so try to put the incident behind you. Like your child, you are only human, and the effects of losing your cool do not last.

6 *Positive action.* Many wonderful parents undertake energetic research into whatever assistance is available, from both the state

and privately, for children with ASD, and what groups or individuals with AS there are in the local area. This can be a big help on the social side. Making friends with other children is important, and the other parents can be a source of understanding, mutual support and sparking of ideas.

It is obvious which response is the most constructive!

It is often said by flummoxed parents that their AS or autistic children 'live in a different world' from the workaday place most ordinary, neurotypical mortals inhabit. Indeed, the writer Charlotte Moore called her piece in the *Guardian* about her autistic sons 'Passport to Another World'. In turn, AS children find it hard to understand 'normal' people and the whole concept of feelings.

It is not surprising that having a child with AS has a marked impact on the parents' relationship with each other, as highlighted by an OASIS survey of 327 parents (see Websites at the end of this book). It can operate equally strongly for better or for worse. Exactly 50 per cent of parents say they get on better – perhaps partly due to the structure imposed by having a diagnosis – while the other half say that things have got worse. Some 25 per cent said they experienced roller-coaster ebbs and flows of feeling about living with an AS child. Fortunately, most couples see eye to eye over important decisions affecting their child, such matters as day-to-day management, medication, education and trying out new ploys. However, two-thirds are aware of extra stress in the marriage, with more arguments, although these are usually resolved in the end.

Janet and Steven

Janet and Steven always discussed the problems and choices that arose with young Stevie, but it was Janet who was generally in charge of the decision-making, while Steven provided extra love, emotional back-up for Janet and the necessary funds. Like more than half the parents in their position, each of them found their partner was their most valuable and effective support.

Something that most couples miss when they have a child with AS is time on their own together as two adults, with this sometimes leading to one of them feeling that he or she is less open emotionally to their partner. Parents may also have problems of their own to contend with, such as (according to the OASIS survey and in order of frequency):

1 Depression.
2 AS (Asperger Syndrome).
3 AD/HD (Attention Deficit/Hyperactivity Disorder).
4 Bipolar disorder, with alternating periods of depression and elation.
5 ASD (Autistic Spectrum Disorder) apart from AS.

The practical effects of having a child with AS disrupt the mother's life more often than the father's. She may be prevented from working outside the home or even entertaining, because she has to devote so much time to the child. This is made worse by the high cost of paying for domestic help to allow her a few hours 'off duty'. Extra expense is often incurred supporting the youngster's special interests – more than 10 per cent of parents find they are spending more than £1,500 annually on books, equipment and courses in this respect.

However, it is important to encourage special interests and knowledge in a child whose confidence is low and has few social skills, and this is an area where parents can indeed make a significant contribution.

Donald
Donald was shy, insignificant-looking and no good at games. He was usually to be seen hanging around forlornly on the edge of a group, with no one letting him join in. Then his parents bought a computer. Donald was fascinated with it and quickly got to know as much as the teacher. He became the acknowledged form-room expert and in great demand among his classmates at school. His confidence rocketed, while his parents played their part by buying him the latest software.

Rivalry between parents, each wanting to be the 'best' and most helpful, may result in the AS youngster feeling overwhelmed. Particularly when there is a major upset, each partner must take the role he does best. With Janet and Steven, for instance, they had found that Janet was better at defusing a crisis like a screaming fit, and Steven's forte was the gentle comforting needed in the aftermath. It is usually better if only one person at a time is doing the talking – or hugging.

Brothers and sisters

Having a brother or sister is often seen as the best thing that can happen to a child with AS. Neurotypical and Asperger children teach each other far better than adults can. A 'normal' sibling can provide an AS youngster with valuable practice in communication and stimulate his imagination. In turn, the neurotypical sibling learns the priceless lessons of tolerance, understanding, patience and responsibility.

Shadowing is a term sometimes used for learning from one another by unconsciously copying what someone else does, and it applies particularly to brothers and sisters. Helpful though it is for a child with AS to have a neurotypical sibling, one danger is that the 'ordinary' youngster will lose out because so much attention is paid to the autistic one. For these 'ordinary' children, quality time with the parents falls to a third of what it was before the arrival and diagnosis of the child with ASD, but some parents, around a quarter, truly believe that they have succeeded in dividing their time and attention equally between their children regardless of disabilities and handicaps.

Children, especially at school, want to be 'just like everyone else', and they are often acutely embarrassed by a sibling with AS who has fits of screaming and other antisocial behaviour. They can be alternately ashamed and jealous over the fuss.

Chloe and Jane

Chloe had always been 'very good' with her younger sister, Jane, who was diagnosed with AS when she was five and a half and Chloe was ten. Jane had been a late talker and walker, and her mother had to wheel her around in a pushchair until she was four. Chloe became very keen on sport, perhaps as a reaction, and won several prizes. When she was twelve she developed anorexia nervosa and her parents spent hours trying to get her to eat. So the situation was reversed: now Chloe was the centre of attention.

Jane showed no ill effects. It seemed as though she were relieved at being out of the spotlight and her behaviour quietened down when she had more time on her own.

Birth order among siblings when one of them has AS has a special effect, whether he is the youngest or the oldest. If the parents have already experienced having a child with AS, naturally they will look out for similar symptoms in their second one. Since no two children with AS are alike, the parents may not recognize a different presentation of the condition. They feel that the second child cannot have AS since he is so unlike his sibling. Of course, it can work the other way. If he resembles what his brother or sister was like at the same stage, there is the advantage of an early diagnosis.

Everard and Nancy

Everard was noisy and destructive – the nursery school could not contain him. He was diagnosed at the age of two and a half, while his sister Nancy, two years older than him, only showed quiet withdrawal to indicate her AS. She was nearly five when it was decided that she also had AS.

Jack and Peter

Jack and Peter both had an exceptional musical ability, but Jack would practise diligently but not excessively, while Peter would repeat the same piece 50 times in his striving for absolute perfection. Peter was considered to have AS because he was also very particular in what he would, and would not, eat; the colours he would accept for his clothes; and the routines with which he ran his day.

Adrian

Adrian, unlike the stereotype of AS children, was a difficult baby and developed into an obstreperous toddler. The doctor suggested that he was a case of ODD – Oppositional Defiant Disorder, which often goes with AS. Adrian remained an only child because his parents felt they could not cope with another child who demanded so much time and attention.

Other parents of AS children did not want bigger families, and others were plagued with infertility problems:

Roger and Mary

Roger had AS, diagnosed when he was already in his twenties. He loved Mary, and because she wanted a baby he struggled with his fear of having sexual intercourse. He was so inhibited that it was difficult for him to complete the act, but on one occasion it worked. Their child was a triumph for Roger and a triumph and a joy to Mary. It seems, so far, that their daughter is unaffected by her father's AS: she is already four years old. They are a happy little family, but Roger does not feel he could go through the sexual side of marriage again.

There are fewer marriages among those with AS, and more of these marriages are childless because of the natural preference for being alone among adults with AS. That being the case, you would expect that the number of people with AS would be falling. However, this is not happening. Of course, with increased knowledge and experience we are diagnosing more cases of AS, but there must be some other factors at work. What advantages are there for those with AS that helps them to thrive? We don't know the answer yet, but we do know that the majority of children with AS feel that they are winners rather than losers in an uphill struggle.

The inside story of AS

The inside story of what it is really like to have a child or children with ASD, either AS or non-specific autism, is entertainingly and graphically told by Charlotte Moore. She is a single mother with three boys; and, as though that were not enough, two of them are autistic. She has published a book, *George and Sam: Autism in the Family*, which describes her extraordinary lifestyle – half nightmare, half comedy – with her three sons. Her story also vividly illustrates the fact that every child is different from every other child, and that every child with AS is different from every other child with AS – even if they are brothers.

Charlotte herself had a conventional middle-class background, with no autistic symptoms in her family. She and her two brothers were rather bookish and had no interest in sport, but they played imaginative games together.

When Charlotte wrote her book, her sons were: 13 (George), 11 (Sam), and 4 (Jake).

George was diagnosed as being autistic when he was three, and Sam at the age of four. Jake showed no sign of autism, but instead all the 'symptoms' of neurotypical normality. The two boys are very different, except that they are particularly beautiful, intelligent-looking children. Physical beauty has often been remarked upon in autistic children. Charlotte's youngest son, Jake, is also attractive. Maybe they all take after their mother.

George is a bundle of nervous energy and has always been excited by the colour red – for example, in a bow on his teddy. He shows the characteristic Asperger trait of particularly acute senses, including smell. He selects his food by sniffing it. Up to the age of two years and three months, he was something of an infant prodigy, enjoying picture books at three months, mastering sit-on toys at six months, and being interested in everything. Just after his second birthday, his phenomenal progress tailed off, but he remained generally bright, very active and easily upset. He was diagnosed as autistic ten years ago, when he was three. ASD was considered uncommon then, and AS was much less recognized than it is today. In fact, Dr Uta Frith had only recently translated Kanner's original research papers from the German. At 13, George had mastered the basic three Rs. He can learn a song quickly and easily, but has no other special talents. He will accept a hug from his mother, but does not return it and never initiates any sign of affection. This is typical of AS.

Sam is two years younger than George. When he was two, and a happy placid child, the psychiatrist confidently reassured Charlotte that there was no need to worry about him being autistic. But when Sam was nearly four, he developed the classic symptoms of autism and became uncommunicative and withdrawn. An educational psychologist pointed out that it was abnormal for Sam to show no interest in puzzles, although he could easily have solved them.

Sam, unlike George, was placid and cheerful, but that did not mean he was no worry. His behaviour was unpredictable. When he was seven he was seen going up to a dog and taking its ball out of its mouth and putting it in his own – a form of shadowing (see page 17). He was always drawing attention to himself by shouting out 'Don't look at me!' when other activities did not work. Sam avoided the limelight and had a disconcerting habit of disappearing – sometimes for hours, and sometimes covering quite a distance. While his mother was frantic with worry, he was unconcerned, as he did not have the imagination to think of the possible dangers.

Jake, the youngest, is, so far, neurotypical. His face beams with delight and he claps his hands when he has a present. He goes to the local primary school, greeting a gang of friends on the way in and entering into all that is going on. What Charlotte appreciates most about him is something her older sons have never done – Jake gives her a casual, quick, parting hug.

George and Sam never played with anyone else or each other. They preferred to play alone or just be alone, not playing. There are some advantages in having a child whose thinking is autistic, demonstrated by Charlotte's two elder sons. They do not squabble or compete with each other, nor complain with the well-worn refrains: 'It isn't fair', 'He started it', or 'It wasn't me'. They don't clamour for the latest – and most expensive – electronic toy, or brand of trainers.

Nothing as simple as that. Because of their skewed thinking, they do things you would never guess. Sam, for instance, startled a local farmer who was having an after-dinner nap by getting into bed with him, wellies and all. George, one evening, decided to join the pigs in their field of mud for a good wallow.

Aside from their odd, unheralded behaviour, Charlotte's boys direct her life by the numerous rituals she has to go through at mealtimes, dressing, bathing, getting ready for school – every part of their daily programme. This seems the only way of getting through the day without tantrums that last for hours, or at least extreme anxiety. Fixations, an overwhelming interest in particular subjects, and obsessions punctuate their days. OCD (Obsessive Compulsive Disorder; see Chapter 7) is a common co-morbid condition in ASD.

To my way of looking at things, Charlotte Moore qualifies for sainthood!

4

The first five years

Mothers used to check their babies for the correct number of fingers and toes. Nowadays, they may be just as anxious about the possibility of ASD or AS. To spot these is by no means as quick and easy as counting to ten. In fact, the subtle signs and symptoms are not definite enough for a diagnosis until the child is about 18 months old. However, the sooner you know if your child is autistic, the sooner you will be able to help him enhance his strengths and cope with his weaknesses, so do always consult your GP if you are worried. A parent's intuition is reliable, so don't allow others, such as medical staff or well-meaning relatives, to fob you off with reassurance that your child is 'fine' if you suspect otherwise.

Normal development – ages and stages

It is only possible to work out where development has gone wrong and is implicated with autism or AS if you have a clear idea of what is normal. Bear in mind that all children, at all stages, are individual and develop according to different timetables.

Brand-new baby

Of course you are thrilled with your brand-new baby. Every tiny detail is terribly important, something to wonder at. You may, though, have a special reason to monitor his development extra closely – for instance, if he has an older brother or sister, or even a distant relative, who has ASD or AS. You will be on the alert for any hint that he has some of the same genes. This is not so that you can 'nip it in the bud' like an illness – his genetic make-up is an unalterable part of your child – but so that you can understand him better.

For the first six weeks your job is to get acquainted with your baby, love him and enjoy him, cuddle him when he cries, croon him a lullaby, tickle his toes and share the cosiness of giving him his feeds. You will be busy.

Three mothers, three babies

Mary, Julie and Shireen made friends in the antenatal clinic and, after straightforward pregnancies and births, promised to keep in touch. Mary and Julie both had boys, John and Richard respectively, while Shireen had a little daughter, Sasha. Each of the mothers, of course, knew that her baby was the best!

Richard, a beautiful baby with clear-cut regular features and delicate complexion, did not cry as much as John, and was not as restless as Sasha. He was a peaceful baby and looked as though he was immersed in his own private thoughts.

By six weeks, all three babies had grown and developed definite personalities. They turned their eyes and heads towards their mother's voice or whatever caught their attention. This was a time when they were learning to love and trust – and bond. When Mary dropped her book on the floor and it made a small bang, John's face crumpled and he began to cry, but she was quickly able to comfort him. By eight weeks, all three had gone through the major experience of discovering their hands – fascinating playthings to watch and bat with. Sasha and John often focused intently on their mothers. 'It's as though he can see right into your soul', said Mary of her John, but Richard seemed to look mostly at the world around him.

By 12 weeks, the babies recognized the important individuals in their lives – Daddy, Granny, and Tig the cat – but they expressed most delight at seeing their mothers, by gurgling and cooing and giving wide, toothless smiles. Richard seemed to take matters more seriously than the others. He accepted cuddles from Julie, but lay in her arms rather stiffly and did not snuggle into them comfortably. He was still fascinated by his hands, and opened and closed his fingers for the pure pleasure of watching their movement.

The first year

What an exciting time, and what huge advances your baby makes in the first 12 months. By the end of this first year, your young hopeful is an eager little explorer, mentally and physically. A big advance is in mobility – crawling, rolling or humping across the floor, fired by the same curiosity that took Christopher Columbus round the globe. Another proud achievement at the age of one is standing upright (although holding on).

Musical appreciation starts now, demonstrated by bouncing to time on his mother's knee or clapping the rhythm as his mother has taught him. He has also learned to use his index finger, usually the right one, to point out something he wants or that you might find interesting. From a rather cautious approach to bath-time as a baby, the toddler now hits the water with his hands and splashes it everywhere.

Even more exciting than his physical progress are his enormous mental advances. The one-year-old has worked out the purpose of everyday articles such as a spoon and fork, brush and comb, or a crayon. Teddy is involved by having his scant fur brushed, or a dolly-sized cup held to his mouth – a matter of imagination. This is something that autistic children are slow to pick up. If Teddy falls on the floor, his 'ordinary' one-year-old owner may kiss him better. This shows empathy, another response that neurotypical 'tinies' learn before the autistic children.

The average one-year-old in Britain knows his name and three proper words – some know many more. Useful words such as 'mine' and 'no' come into play early on, and a group of anatomical terms – nose, eye, finger, toe, etc. – come particularly easily to boys.

Language, like teeth, appears through a built-in, genetically controlled programme, separate from other aspects of development. The word-store at 18 months may vary between 2 and 200, and autistic children are likely to be at either extreme. Repetitive phrases like *eeny*, *meeny*, *miney*, *mo*, or *fee*, *fi*, *fo*, *fum* are an enjoyable step in learning the rhythm of language and poetry, and autistic children sometimes chant them over and over. Language problems are common in AS people, and some with autistic traits are slow to speak. Einstein was one such.

First-year milestones

Every single baby is unique, and John, Richard and Sasha, mentioned above, were no exceptions. John was the muscle man, Sasha the socialite, and Richard the thinker of the group. None of them was 'average' (there is no such child), but they were all travelling in the same direction, each at his own pace. On the way, they will pass some milestones, again at their individual times:

- 6 months: holds up arms, ready to be picked up; excited to see mother, cries or looks sad if she goes away; friendly to everyone.
- 9 months: says *da*, *ma*, *ba* and *ll*, just as single-syllable babbling sounds.

- 10 months: one real, meaningful word; in Sasha's case, this was *No*. The word *mine* came soon after.
- 11 months: says *Mama* and *Dada* as appropriate, and three proper words.
- 1 year: walking (John started walking at 10 months); shows sympathy, affection – and guilt; imaginative play with bear or truck or dolly-size cups and equipment; points to draw your attention to what he wants you to see; suddenly shy of strangers; copies adults' expressions (e.g. putting out his tongue); 6 to 20 words, also learned by imitation (needs to hear a word 500 times to learn it).

What to watch for:

As I have said, it is hard to diagnose AS during this period, but possible warning signs at this stage include a general lack of social interaction, such as no 'social' smiles; no facial expressions to show feelings, such as delight or fear; or lack of eye contact. Your baby's attention is not attracted to Mother or any other person; and he ignores what is going on around him or any people present. Babbling, which typically develops around six months, is absent.

Older baby and toddler – up to three years

Richard

It was when Richard, whom we mentioned earlier, was between nine and 18 months old that Julie began to get worried. The other toddlers were beginning to socialize, play near other children, and look at what they were doing. Soon they were sharing a game and their imagination was sparked off by each other's activities. Cars crashed and dolls were frequently put to bed in a shoebox.

In contrast, Richard played by himself. He made no attempt to link up with another child. Sometimes he would spend half an hour repeating the same sequence of movements with a toy or some other object that had caught his eye.

Looking back, it became clear that from day one Richard's behaviour was different from that of ordinary, neurotypical babies. He had taken no more interest in his mother than in anybody else – or a chair. Richard's general lack of social concern and his attitude of detachment persisted all through his earliest weeks, months and years. He did not 'alert' to the sound of his mother's voice and he avoided eye contact, nor did he try to communicate by such body language as frowning and other facial expressions.

The period of 18 months to three years is supremely important. It holds the key to the diagnosis of Kanner's classic type of autism, the wider concept of ASD, and sometimes a hint of AS specifically.

This is a time of blossoming social skills. By the age of two, the child enjoys the company of peers, and by three he may play with them. Imagination and other cognitive skills take off – for example, imaginative play and make-believe games such as tea parties. Autistic and AS children often miss out on this. Sometimes they tell other people about fantastic adventures they have had, but they do not really believe in them. Imaginary friends crop up with both neurotypical and autistic youngsters, especially only children, as so many autistic children are.

Up to the age of two, young children develop fears of wild animals, strangers, being left all by themselves . . . and the dark. In later years, it is social situations that make them nervous, especially AS youngsters.

Major physical advances apply equally to neurotypical and children with ASD during this time. At 15 months, the toddler can stand firmly on two feet, and when he is three he can balance on one leg for a few dizzy seconds. Small precision skills, such as picking up tiny beads, are easily mastered by neurotypical toddlers by this age. Autistic children are frequently clumsy over big movements, but may show skill with more delicate ones.

Eighteen to 30 months is the period for tantrums, and this is more likely to be extreme for the autistic child because he has more reason than neurotypical children to feel anxiety and frustration. The tantrum is the result of an all-out effort to make himself understood when his thinking runs along different lines from other people's.

Milestones between the ages of one and three

- 18 months:
  Vocabulary includes *eyes*, *nose*, *toes* and other parts of the body, and may reach 200 words.
  Manual dexterity – can build a tower of three or four bricks.
  Likes looking at a picture book on his mother's knee for two or three minutes.
- 2 years:

Word-store increasing to 300 or more. Two- or three-word sentences.

Manual dexterity – can build a tower of six or seven bricks.

Plays make-believe games – for instance, driving a racing car or making tea.

Socializing – likes to play near other children, sometimes with them.

Can do 'round and round' scribbling with a crayon.

Can kick a ball with a stiff, straight leg.

- 3 years:

Up to 1,000 words in three- to four-word sentences.

Comments leading to conversation.

Makes a 'train' with up to nine bricks.

Hand skills – uses a spoon and fork, holds a pencil the right way, and copies a cross and a circle.

What to watch for:

Impaired communication may show up as slow development of language, especially comprehension; for example, no separate words by 18 months; no two-word phrases by 24 months – for example, 'good boy', 'not nice', 'all gone'. A particular sign is loss of words or meaningful gestures previously known (see Regression, below). Your child may show a lack of response to his name. He may have poor body language such as pointing, holding arms up to be lifted, smiling, holding out a toy to show and share.

Impaired social skills may include a poor ability to imitate other people's actions, such as clapping hands; a lack of interest in other children – for example, he is never the one to start play with another child. He may lack empathy, with no apparent awareness of happiness, laughter, distress or tears in another person; he may not greet or even show that he recognizes someone he knows.

Regression

Regression, or going backwards in development, is a particular feature of AS and can be one of the most upsetting symptoms for parents who have assumed that their child is developing normally.

In his second year, Richard – one of the three children we

---

looked at above – stopped using as many words as he had done before. To take another example, Tony and David had been developing at the same pace throughout their first year, and both had achieved a vocabulary of ten or more words. But while Tony went from strength to strength, David's progress came to a halt. A few weeks later, he seemed to be going in reverse. Two of the phrases he had recently acquired were apparently lost: he was just 22 months old. Then he began to progress again, haltingly.

Regression is the term for this loss of ground. It affects 25–30 per cent of children who turn out to have AS, between the ages of 15 and 21 months. Another period of regression, affecting 7–8 per cent of the children, comes on after the age of two. Not only are speech and language affected, but the youngster withdraws socially, losing eye contact and his interest in the outside world.

In some cases, a child who is regressing changes his sleeping and eating habits and starts new ones – for instance, hand-flapping or non-stop humming. A careful review of the child's early development often reveals that it was not as straightforward as it seemed – for example, he may not have understood the meaning of common metaphors and slang, although he used the words.

The pre-school child – three to five years

Up to and into their third year, Sasha and John (mentioned on page 23) continued to develop socially, enjoying the company of other children and showing sympathy if one of them had a tumble. They were fast becoming chatterboxes, and beginning to have special friends. Their mothers asked them to each other's houses for tea. Sasha had three friends to her third birthday party and they played games like ring o' roses.

This is a time of accelerating social development, with children enjoying co-operative play and perhaps loosely organized group games (such as duck-duck-goose). The child's growing independence shows in an increased ability to dress himself, wash and dry his face – and sometimes in defiance as he tests his freedom and abilities. His motor development becomes more sophisticated and he may jump, skip and hop with increasing dexterity, in contrast to the AS child who may remain clumsy. Fine motor development also blooms, and he may master scissors and the art of drawing an increasingly recognizable object.

Many rising fives are now looking forward to starting school, with all its social thrills and challenges.

Pre-school milestones:

- Highly sociable.
- Chatters and asks endless questions.
- Answers questions and tells simple stories.
- Word-store of up to 2,000 words or more.
- Highly imaginative.
- By the age of five, prints letters and draws recognizable shapes.
- May tie shoelaces.
- Right- or left-handedness established.
- Jumps, hops, skips.
- Can ride a scooter.

It was when he was nearly four that Mary noticed that her John was usually on the edge of a group of friends. He preferred to be alone and avoided playing with more than one child at a time. Nor did he have a friend – that is, any child he specially liked or who liked him. It was at about this age that John developed an intense interest in radio stations all over the world, including their wavelengths and time zones. Instead of chattering with another child as part of his play, John began to talk in a flat, monotonous, pedantic voice, always about radio stations. He did not pay much attention to what other people said, even about 'his' subject unless it was an adult giving him some information. He did not look at the people he was talking to, nor back up his words with gestures or facial expressions. He was exceedingly long-winded and boring, so other children did not want to be friends with him. There had been so much publicity about AS that Mary quickly found enough about it on the internet to suspect that John had AS.

What to watch for:
Impaired communication may now manifest as abnormal language or having no language, or odd patterns of speech such as *echolalia* – that is a repetition of words or questions he has just heard. Sometimes this is done to clarify them (for instance, if he is asked 'Would you like an apple?' he may reply, 'Would I like an apple?'

or just repeat 'an apple'). He may reverse pronouns, referring to himself as *you*, *she* or *he*. He may also have an unusual choice of words, frequently stilted, old-fashioned or inappropriately adult; or his speech may be restricted to a few 'favourite' topics.

Social impairment may show up as preferring solitary pastimes to imaginative activities with others, especially repetitive play, such as turning switches on and off, or lining up toys, showing a limitation of interests, activities and range of behaviour. If he does join in with the play of others, he does so inappropriately – for instance, with aggression, or spoiling the game. If he has started school, he may be unaware of how to behave in class, appearing uncooperative with the teacher, and he does not follow school fashions in clothes, speech, behaviour or interests. He cannot stand up for himself, may show an obstinate refusal to be hurried, and may ignore adults and being scolded. He may be abnormally sensitive to sound or touch, as though they actually cause pain. He may show an extreme reaction to any invasion of his personal space, and cannot tolerate change.

Diagnosis

Julie, and her rather introverted husband, Mark, a computer buff, decided to consult a child psychiatrist about Richard's worrying withdrawal and regression in vocabulary. She advised them that their son was almost certainly a classic autistic.

AS is regarded by some people as 'high-functioning autism', but most parents and workers consider it a specific and separate condition within the autistic spectrum. Initially, however, a diagnosis of autism can be reliably made between the ages of two and three, and this is almost synonymous with ASD for practical purposes.

There is no definitive test, so the diagnosis depends on observing the child's behaviour, with special enquiries made about the key features as laid out in Kanner's checklist (see Chapter 1; see also the Appendix at the end of this book).

Many of the characteristics of AS overlap with those of autism, but tend to emerge later, sometimes not until puberty; but language and learning difficulties are less common.

Checklist for Asperger Syndrome (AS)

Impaired social interaction shown by at least two of the following:

- Poor non-verbal communication – that is, eye contact, facial expression, posture or gestures.
- Does not relate to other children at the usual age.
- No spontaneous sharing of pleasure or something interesting.
- Inappropriate or absent responses to social or emotional approaches – for instance, laughs at something sad.
- Preoccupation with one or more special interests.
- Talks pedantically with adult vocabulary and grammar.
- Does not understand that other people have feelings, and cannot express his own.
- Cannot generalize from one event – for instance, that it is safer to cross the road with an adult.
- Resists any change, even going from one room to another; keeps to the same routine.

(*Note regarding play*: There is a choice of checklists or diagnostic indices for AS: American, British/European and Australian. The last one puts play at the top of the list – that is, that youngsters with AS do not understand how to play with others. This might seem unimportant, but it is the very essence of being a child – or even a puppy! For example, it should always ring alarm bells when a school-age child (nursery or primary school) routinely chooses to stay inside and look at a book during playtime.)

A variety of cases

The following all illustrate what a variety of forms AS may take:

- *Graham* only began to show signs of autism at the age of three, when he started nursery school. Other AS children cannot cope when they meet the stress of 'big' school, after nursery school. They may behave normally while they are in school, but break down into an anxiety state, or an angry outburst, when they are safely at home. It can also work in reverse. A teacher who is used to dealing with autism may save the situation or, as a last resort, home education offers a temporary rescue package.

- *John* is an only child. Because he spent so much time with grown-ups, he had a good vocabulary, and his parents, Granny and aunties all thought he was particularly clever. Children of his own age thought he was thick. As there had always been an adult on hand, John did not master such skills as buttons and zips – also, he was no good at ball games. Clumsiness added to John's difficulties. What made matters worse was that the adults, including his teacher, 'knew' he was bright and put it down to laziness when his shoelaces were dragging along undone and his jacket done up on the wrong button. He was chronically anxious.

  Then John's mother, who read all she could about bringing up children, came across an article about Asperger Syndrome and the three-year lag in development up to the age of 19 compared with other children. John's mother recognized his difficulties – he was still functioning at age seven when he was chronologically ten. She no longer criticized his mistakes, but helped him practise such skills as buttoning his cuffs or sharpening a pencil. John reacted with a reduction in the number of his anxiety attacks.

- *Ronnie* collects adults' peculiar sayings – for example, saying that someone is a 'snake in the grass', although he is indoors and is a person, not a reptile. Another one is that they are 'as cross as two sticks' and the very horrible one about 'more than one way to skin a cat'. Ronnie finds these sayings confusing, but is very proud of his own jokes. He links the proverb 'pigs might fly' with 'pie in the sky' with a long explanation about pigs enjoying eating pie. He is surprised that no one laughs.

- *Gareth*, at three and a half, was doing well at nursery school until it came to writing his name. He had a junior form of dyslexia. The letter G was a tricky one, and he refused to go any further. He was not a sociable child and preferred to stay indoors at break, looking at a book, in spite of his teacher's exhortations to go out and play 'in the lovely fresh air'. She came back into the classroom one day to find Gareth engrossed with her laptop. He was already banging out a few words. From then on, while his handwriting improved at a snail's-pace, he soon learned to communicate expertly through the keyboard – a shining example of the fact that Aspies often develop their IT skills much sooner than neurotypical children.

Other diagnoses to consider

General learning disability may be difficult to distinguish from autism in the very young, but it is assessed as occurring in 75 per cent of children with ASD. However, this is probably an over-estimate because of problems with regard to writing in otherwise bright children.

Language disorder

This may show up in a difficulty in talking with and relating to others of the same age, and a lack of imaginative play.

Other specific developmental disorders

For instance, poor co-ordination and clumsiness, Rett's disorder and other rare neurological disorders.

Reactions to stress

For instance, rows at home, illness.

Medical assessment

This is part of looking out for autism. It requires:

- a detailed history of development, noting any deviations from normal;
- a physical examination, along with routine hearing and vision tests;
- blood tests to check for levels of lead, anaemia, fragile X chromosome, thyroid hormone.

Associated problems

Epilepsy

About 17 per cent of autistic youngsters have seizures either in early childhood or adolescence. This is a lower number than was previously thought, but still nearly double the neurotypical count.

Psychiatric problems

Likewise, about 17 per cent of autistic youngsters suffer from problems such as depression, anxiety, sleeping and eating disorders, and OCD (Obsessive Compulsive Disorder). Children with autism run twice the risk of these problems occurring compared with those with learning difficulties.

Bowel function

This problem occurring in those with autism is currently the subject of research, harking back to the time when the MMR vaccine was thought to cause Crohn's disease as well as autism.

5

School-time

School age is a golden period for many, if not most, children. This is when a child takes his momentous first step out of the nest and into the world of school where another lady, not Mummy, calls the shots and knows everything.

Starting school is a huge event in any child's life, whether they be 'ordinary' or AS. It involves a gigantic leap into a completely new world, with its characteristic sounds, sights and smells. Every child is excited and anxious on that first day, but youngsters with AS find it doubly traumatic since even the smallest change is alien to their nature. Sameness gives them a sense of security and that vanishes like a puff of smoke in the new environment.

Most neurotypical children focus on the social aspect of their new life – break, school meals and games. Lessons figure low on the list of what is important for most of them, but not for a child like John, whom we met in the last chapter (page 32). He preferred sitting quietly, listening to the teacher if the subject interested him and he could understand the point of it. He liked maths best because he could rely on it making sense, but poetry seemed a meaningless jumble of words. Sasha (see page 23), being an extravert, settled into school easily and soon had two best friends. Her favourite subjects, she said, were English (stories) and netball, but she often 'forgot' her homework. She was a well-adjusted 'neurotypical schoolie'.

Screaming, tantrums, hitting out or biting are AS-type reactions to the overwhelming emotional stress, and school is fraught with problems for AS children. Some of these problems are rooted in the school set-up and the difficulties this produces in the child himself. There is also the impact of the teacher and the other children on the 'new boy' to contend with.

Hardly any adults with AS say that they enjoyed their time at school. The three worst features are often homework, team games and break-times. School lunches and travelling in the school bus are also dreaded. Except for homework, these are all occasions when there is an opportunity for teasing (or worse) by other children, when the teacher's attention is occupied elsewhere.

Geoffrey

Geoffrey had been given to racing round the house every now and again making whooping noises. When he was five and had to go to school, he found it frustrating to have to stay in one place, without talking, through a whole lesson. Then, when he had got used to sitting there, everyone would be uprooted to go to another classroom or the gym. It made him anxious not knowing what would come next and reorientating himself each time. The racket of the other children between lessons and at break, laughing and shrieking, banging their desks and stampeding along the corridor, hurt his ears, and confused and frightened him. He was particularly sensitive to loud noise. These interludes, which the other children loved, were his least favourite aspect of school – apart from sport.

Even when Geoffrey got home, the spirit of school still bugged him in the form of homework – just when he wanted to escape into the quiet of his own room and his personal world of solving maths puzzles and working out new ones. His mother, who was a far better organizer than Geoffrey, took matters in hand, allowing him half an hour for homework immediately after tea. After this, he could do what he liked until supper. She hoped he would go out and play with friends, but Geoffrey did not make any friends at school. Although he would answer politely if anyone asked him an easy – that is, factual – question, he did not know how to talk to the other children in an ordinary relaxed way.

This resulted in him being left out of the other children's games. Once he tried to join in with a group, screwing up his courage to ask if he might play too, but they told him to go away. School team games were even more humiliating. They involved everyone being picked for one side or the other, but Geoffrey was invariably left until last. Whichever team he was finally allocated to, they groaned 'Do we have to have him?'

School activities

Team games are a recipe for destroying self-confidence in children with AS, but they do better in sports that depend on individual effort rather than co-operation with others. Such activities include running, swimming, ski-ing, skating, gym, athletics and marathons – none of them freely available in most schools. In fact, most children with AS are not greatly drawn to healthy physical exercise with other people, but prefer 'brain work' by themselves, especially when it involves their self-chosen special interest.

Maths, music, astronomy and scientific subjects such as chemistry, physics and computer technology can often become an AS youngster's obsession, his special subject. Prehistory and dinosaurs have a particular fascination for some children. In fact, it is estimated that 100 per cent of children with AS have one or more absorbing interests! They may become recognized experts in the classroom or the whole school, or even when they are adults.

Like a large proportion of children with AS, Geoffrey was hopeless at throwing, kicking and especially catching a ball, so he did a lot of standing about. The sports teacher told him to 'snap out of it and pull his socks up'. He might just as well have spoken in Dutch for all the sense his words meant to Geoffrey. What had his socks got to do with anything? Where Geoffrey really flourished was during a quiet evening at his hobby of maths puzzles.

Language difficulties

Language difficulties, particularly frequent in the families of AS children, may show up for the first time at school.

Laurence

Laurence found it difficult to open a conversation or join in when other people were talking. It always came as an unwelcome interruption. Although he was comfortable with answering plain questions with unequivocal answers, he often could not make head or tail of metaphors, jokes, sarcasm or idiom. Trying to express his own emotions was another problem, and this led to him having difficulties in understanding and empathizing with other people's feelings. Seeing another person's point of view is one of the basic bricks for making a relationship.

AS is a physical disorder in development, often in a part of the brain that deals with language, and language difficulties in general are more common in families with any form of ASD. Problems that can result include *dyslexia, dyspraxia, dysgraphia* and *dyscalculia*. All these conditions are variations of development and have a physical basis, not an emotional or psychological one.

Dyslexia

This is the most common disorder, affecting 15–20 per cent of school-age children, with many, but not all, of them having AS. It consists of difficulties in reading, writing and spelling. Although no one can remove this tiny developmental abnormality, coaching and practice can improve the symptoms almost to vanishing point. The distinguished politician Lord Heseltine is one of the success stories.

Dyspraxia

This is similarly caused, but affects muscle co-ordination and movement. The effects are clumsiness and difficulties in such everyday activities as using a knife and fork or getting dressed. Geoffrey's 'butter-fingers' were a symptom of dyspraxia, while some dyspraxic children have an odd gait.

Dysgraphia

This involves drawing, including the formation of letters. A child with AS may make the most beautiful, detailed drawings and yet have a dislike of writing and may avoid even taking notes in a lesson. Dysgraphia, dyslexia and dyspraxia can all contribute to the notoriously large, untidy handwriting that teachers complain about with AS pupils.

Dyscalculia

This is a similar kind of problem, but it affects arithmetic. The youngster has difficulty in grasping the whole concept of numbers. This usually surprises the adults because there are some AS children who hit the headlines with their mathematical skills, taking A level algebra at the age of nine. This is exceptional, even in AS.

Bullying

The problem that causes the maximum unhappiness to the maximum number of school-age AS children is bullying. Luke Jackson, the young author of *Freaks, Geeks and Asperger Syndrome*, is one of them, and he adds the dimension of time to the grim picture. 'All my life I have been bullied,' he writes, explaining for the sake of his super-logical readers with AS that he does not mean non-stop, but frequently over time. Bullies never give up. With Luke it started at nursery school and continued throughout the school years.

How can you tell a bully? There are two main clues:

1 He says or does things that hurt you even if he is pretending to be nice.
2 He usually has two or three friends with him, but chooses opportunities when you are by yourself.

Bullies are cowards and do everything to keep themselves out of trouble and to blame others. The effect, naturally enough, is to make the person feel anxious and miserable, and sometimes scared. Since most bullying takes place at school or travelling to and from it, children who have been tormented there will get to dread it. Teachers pick up the bad vibes without knowing where they come from and say the youngsters are 'difficult'.

There are several kinds of bullying:

Verbal bullying

This means calling the victim names like *freak*, *Mummy's pet*, *nerd* or *anorak* and saying hurtful things about him or his family, or even his cat. These may be obviously rude or sneakily facetious, so that it takes a moment or two to realize that he is being got at. Facetious remarks are intended to be funny – except to the victim – and often sound as though they mean the opposite of what they say, such as 'Aren't you clever?' when the child has just made a silly mistake or accidentally dropped something. Bullies make personal remarks about their victim's clothes, hairstyle or size. 'Fatty' is a favourite epithet.

Mimicking the way a person talks or walks, so that everybody laughs at him and makes him feel stupid, is a particularly nasty sort of bullying.

Physical bullying

There are 100 ways of doing this and it seems as though bullies try them all. A lot of AS people are especially sensitive to being touched and it may actually cause them pain. Therefore a bully can upset a vulnerable victim with very little effort, and may resort to pushing, shoving the unlucky person out of a queue, pinching and hitting him, or stamping on his toe. Tripping someone up on purpose, and the even more dangerous trick of taking his chair away just as he is about to sit on it, are great sport for the bully.

Other bully tactics are slamming a door in his face, shouting

'Sorry!' at the same time, or 'accidentally' bumping into him when he is carrying a loaded dinner tray or a hot drink. Then there is pulling a small strand of hair, which is more painful than tugging at a handful. Girls are most at risk. One AS girl I knew sat in front of a bully at school and he tried to set her hair alight with a cigarette lighter he'd got that looked like a tiny gun. Poking the victim through the back of his chair is another of the small actions that the teacher may not notice or may assume was accidental.

Secondhand bullying

This also comes in two types. The verbal kind means saying nasty things about the victim to other people, spreading rumours, and telling tales that are often lies, to get him into trouble. The physical sort of secondhand bullying involves attacks on his property – like hiding his ruler or set square, taunting him by holding it just out of his reach, or even throwing it out of the window. His school books may be scribbled on and his homework turns up dirty and crumpled on the floor. The teacher blames him. Finally, his lunchbox looks as though someone has sat on it. On one occasion, an AS boy found an earthworm in with his food, and occasionally possessions are actually stolen.

Silent bullying

This is one of the most cruel forms, and girls especially use it to hurt a victim without it being obvious to the authorities.

Mervyn

Mervyn moved up into the second class when he was six. He was the youngest and smallest in the class and he was always being pushed out of the way, so he told his teacher. She, in turn, told the other children that they ought to be nice to anyone new. (Mervyn was the only new boy.) Four or five of them sent him to Coventry (they did not speak to him or answer if he spoke), and talked about him loudly to one another, saying he was a sneak and a tell-tale. The teacher did not realize what was happening. In the end, the bullies got bored with it and gave up.

Helping your child understand bullying

Parents can help by making sure that their child understands what is meant by bullying in all its aspects.

Tim

Tim was the smallest boy in his class and he had to wear pebble-thick glasses because he was short-sighted. He also had AS, so he was even more different from the others. He did not have any friends, but did not know why, except that nobody liked him. This made him sad and he sometimes cried privately after a day at school. When his mother asked him, Tim always said that no one was bullying him. This was partly because he did not understand what bullying could entail. His mum had asked him about pushing and punching and pinching, and he said quite truthfully that this was not happening.

What he did not know was that one of the nastiest forms of bullying is non-stop sneaky harassment. For instance, ink got spilt all over his exercise book, the choc bar always disappeared from his lunchbox, his homework went missing, and his blazer button came off. All these things happened out of the teacher's earshot or eyeshot. Tim tried keeping out of sight of the big boys in quiet corners, or hanging about near an adult.

Tim's parents had always fooled themselves that he was perfectly ordinary – just a bit shy. Luckily, as it turned out, a new family moved in next door with a son of Tim's age who had been diagnosed AS.

Neither of the boys knew how to mix with others, but their parents palled up and joined a local parents' group for disabled children. It meant that there was always help, advice and empathy on tap. They found that being the parent of an Aspie was like joining a huge extended family. Everyone agreed that the worst thing that can happen to an AS child, and one of the most common, is to be the victim of covert bullying. It follows only too easily from being misunderstood and looking at things differently from other children – for example, having no interest in football or other team games and preferring their own company to anyone else's.

Teachers

While teachers usually want to be friendly, large class sizes often mean they cannot get to know all the children. This puts a strain on their patience. A teacher under stress may take it out on a kid who is obviously bright, but seems to misunderstand deliberately. This is bullying, too.

My friend Clive is a schoolteacher in a big comprehensive with special responsibility for children who are – horrible word – failing.

It means they are having difficulties at school, and a common difficulty is being the victim of bullies. He finds that AS youngsters are bullied much more than those who are physically handicapped, have serious learning difficulties or severe autism. Other people feel vaguely threatened by a child who is different in a way they cannot pinpoint. To be singled out by the teacher for any reason, even for praise, can draw the attention of a bully looking for someone to hurt.

Reggie

Reggie had been born with cerebral palsy and had a limp. He also had AS. This made him an easy victim: a little different from the other boys, and you could see that he wouldn't be able to run away. He only had a short walk home, just past one corner of a road with little gardens at the front of the houses. The bully was a big boy called Fred, the leader of a gang of three. They would get ahead of Reggie, wait round the corner and, when he came along, snatch his school cap off him and throw it into the nearest garden. The lady whose garden it was became cross when he knocked on the door to ask if he could get his cap – for the third time. The other boys had always disappeared by then.

The business of the cap became a regular event. Reggie was not hurt physically although he felt under threat, but the cap was looking the worse for wear, so that his teacher said it was a disgrace. The bullies said they would beat Reggie up if he 'told'. So he did not tell anyone. The good thing that happened was that one of the big boys, a prefect, saw what they were doing and reported the bullies to the head. That put a stop to their games for a while, but they started up again within a few weeks. Dealing with bullies requires patience and persistence – and courage.

Helping your child deal with bullying

Teach your child strategies for dealing with bullies:

- Try teaching your child to avoid the problem in advance: ask him to stay near an adult, preferably – but not essentially – one whom he knows. Bullies don't like anyone important seeing what they are doing. When bullying is actually happening, your child can ask for help from any adult in sight.
- Suggest that for now he tries to avoid being alone – for instance, at break or when walking home from school. Now is a good time

for him to work at making some friends, even if he likes being alone.

- Encourage your child to actively avoid a known bully or someone he doesn't trust. If confronted by a bully, he can adopt a casual look, or walk away briskly – not running.
- If the worst happens and he does suffer bullying, try to encourage him to keep a stiff upper lip during the event – explain that crying only rewards and encourages the bully.
- Your child can also work at keeping fit or taking up a martial art so that his reaction times are spot on, no one can catch him unawares, and he can defend himself if necessary. Taekwondo is popular among those with AS because its principles stress defending the weak rather than injuring an opponent.
- Try to ensure your child tells someone if he has been, or is being, bullied. Try to get across to him the importance of not suffering in silence: bullying does not get better by itself. He may need reassurance that bullying is not his fault.
- Discourage him from using tactics such as hitting back, trading insults, or trying to be a bully himself. AS people aren't nasty enough to succeed in this.
- Try to find out if any uninformed adults have been telling him that bullying is inevitable and that it is good for a youngster to 'learn to stand up for himself'. This is nonsense and should be exposed as such.

Home schooling: the ultimate educational choice

Knowledge, like food, is only nourishing if it is absorbed. A child takes nothing in while he is suffering agonies of fear. At school he is like an alien in a foreign country. The noise and the number of other children contrast with the quiet, safe, familiarity of home with Mum, where he is understood and helped with the really difficult things. For the AS child, these things are making contact with other people, communicating with them, and making head or tail of what they say and do.

Martin
Martin was eight, the nadir of a child's self-confidence, and he had just moved classes. He began picking his skin until it bled, and twiddling his hair until he had made a bald patch, but he

managed to suppress his more violent feelings at school. It was when he went home and relaxed his control that he fell apart, with terrible tantrums, screaming and smashing his toys. He cried long into the night every night. Some children react the opposite way, and are happy enough at home, but overwhelmed by panic at school.

While the school was geared up to help with academic difficulties, it offered no support with the social hurdles that an AS child like Martin had to overcome. It was clear that he was a constant irritation to the teacher and strained her patience. For Martin's part, he was doing his best to be helpful and could not understand why he was always being punished. For instance, as his best subject was maths, when they were doing a test in class he would reel off the correct answers while the other children were laboriously working them out. Then there was his apparently deliberate misunderstanding of instructions. When the teacher said 'Now go to page 9' after the children had completed an exercise on page 8, Martin merely turned the page while the others busily did the exercise. 'But she didn't say . . .' he said. Other children soon notice if a teacher lets her irritation show, and tend to copy her attitude. The scene is then set for the bullies. Martin's mother went to see the teacher, but this only made matters worse. One of the other boys recognized her, and a group of them jeered at Martin as a baby and tell-tale. This became a regular sport.

It was at this juncture that Martin's parents felt they must rescue him from this daily misery. They decided to remove him from school and teach him at home. Their first task was to research the legal situation.

The law with regard to home education

No one *has* to go to school, but parents have a duty to ensure that their child receives adequate education in the years of compulsory schooling: from the age of five to sixteen. This would be more accurately termed *compulsory education.*

Children's right to education

The Education Act 1996 states that parents (or their equivalent) are responsible for their child's efficient, full-time education, suitable for:

1 Their age, ability and aptitude.

2 Any Special Educational Needs (SEN).

This must be provided *either* by regular attendance at school *or* 'otherwise'. 'Otherwise' is the key word.

Parents have rights too

The Human Rights Act 2000 makes it clear that no person shall be denied the right to education. The state shall respect the right of parents to ensure that such education and teaching is in conformity with their own religious and philosophical convictions.

The law is no barrier to education at home, but it is a huge commitment and requires courage and enthusiasm, usually mainly from the mother, although any input from the father is worth its weight in gold. As we have seen, most AS children are boys, whose natural interests are likely to be in scientific subjects and computers. Four-year-olds are often computer-literate today, sometimes by-passing the acquisition of handwriting skills.

The youngster having home schooling can join or rejoin the mainstream educational system at any time.

Children going into mainstream education have to register by the time they are five, and the parents of those opting out must inform the authorities and explain their alternative plan. The parent who is going to teach the child herself does not require a teaching or other formal teaching qualification.

Reasons for choosing home education

- The child is not emotionally ready to start school.
- He may have suffered a recent trauma – for instance, parents' divorce, death of grandmother, change of school class.
- He is showing signs of stress in his behaviour (as Martin did with skin-picking).
- He is consistently unhappy.
- His parents are opposed to the kind of education on offer by the state.
- Persistent bullying.
- Teacher or school out of sympathy with AS.
- 'Too gifted for the school' – this is sometimes a parent's wishful thinking.

The downside of home education

- Money: a mother cannot go out and earn when she is acting as her child's teacher. On top of this, books and equipment are required and these can be costly.
- Missing out on socialization; that is, mixing with other children, learning to play and make friends (see below).
- Life is complicated if one child goes to school and the other does not – a timetable like Spaghetti Junction!

The tasks involved in home schooling

When a child is not attending regular school, the responsibility for his social life falls on to his mother. It means taking every opportunity for him to be with other children: special clubs, classes and courses, such as music and dancing, handicrafts, art, Saturday and holiday workshops, swimming ... and a load more. (See the section under Useful Addresses, at the end of this book, with regard to home schooling.)

Planning the 'non-school' day can be difficult. While there is freedom to construct a flexible timetable it is best to work out some guidelines. The time spent on 'school' should be roughly equivalent to school hours: say, three hours in the morning and two hours in the afternoon, with two 15-minute breaks, and opportunities for fresh air and exercise. Homework becomes a special project that the student works on alone and then shows the 'teacher'. There is no compulsion to follow the National Curriculum, but there are advantages to doing so. The books are freely available, BBC programmes and CD-ROMs are based on it, and it also makes it easy to go back into mainstream schooling as some youngsters do in the later stages of their education, and when they feel able to cope.

6

The Teenage Years

Puberty is often late in children with ASD, both physically and psychologically. Children with AS develop in slow and sometimes painful steps mentally, emotionally and, most of all, socially. For them, puberty ushers in a long learning phase of adolescence, years longer than in neurotypical children. It is not unusual for an AS youngster to have his first date at 19 or 20, with sexual interest and thoughts of marriage postponed to the mid-thirties.

Few AS youngsters make the spectacular bodily changes that characterize some of their neurotypical peers – which often seem to happen almost overnight. It is rare to see an AS teenager towering over his classmates or having an early interest in sex. The physical developments bring with them extreme self-consciousness. This is more acute for autistic and other special youngsters than for neurotypical ones. The drive towards independence, an important part of growing up, is a threat rather than a thrill to the AS adolescent with his dread of change, and makes it difficult for him to fit in with other children. The physical/emotional upheaval of puberty may also lead to disconcerting changes in a youngster's behaviour, leaving his parents flummoxed.

The late start in growing up means that an AS youngster who looks old enough to be emotionally mature is likely to be incredibly naïve and at risk of being exploited, sexually and otherwise, including through the questionable blessing of the internet. Not only do they develop slowly, but young people with AS tend to have a touchingly childlike moral outlook often unaffected by the principles and beliefs of their streetwise peers in school and the outside world.

They want to do what is right and correct rather than grabbing all they can get from our consumerist world. Loyalty and honesty – and, especially, telling the truth – are second nature to them. Their parents will have stressed the virtues of kindness and politeness, as parents always do. This puts the ethos of the teenager with AS a million miles away from that of the many materially minded neurotypical adolescents, and makes him liable to their jeering. The agonizing shyness all teenagers experience is exaggerated in an AS youngster because he really is different, with his extra sensitivity to touch, sight and sound, and also his great difficulty in understanding what other people feel, and what they mean by their slangy words. 'Cool' and 'wicked', for example, express approval in teen-speak, but to a literally minded AS child they describe temperature and bad behaviour respectively.

The importance of knowing the diagnosis

This opens the door to mutual understanding and usually has a positive effect. Most children say that they wish they had known earlier that they were AS: 64 per cent of the parents in the OASIS survey tell their children that they have AS within a year of hearing the diagnosis themselves.

Most parents tell their children that they have AS, and what that means, when they are about six, the age for asking questions. The explanation, hopefully, expresses the concept that AS is a gift and a privilege, not a disease. It is an integral part of the youngster's nature and therefore permanent – and it involves a difficulty in understanding neurotypical people whose brains work differently. They are a constant puzzle to the AS children who use words, including long ones, with dictionary correctness, and apply simple logic to what they do. By contrast, neurotypical adults and children use words in a more random fashion, to mean what they want them to mean. There is a kind of imaginative guesswork from the context instead of applying the literal meaning.

In metaphorical phrases, the AS teenager needs to understand both types of meaning and sometimes has to learn by heart the underlying neurotypical meanings of common sayings such as 'It's a long lane that has no turning' or 'It's no use crying over spilt milk', and logical thinking can sometimes get a youngster with AS into trouble.

Adrian again
Adrian got into hot water – one of the expressions that would have puzzled him – for refusing to do a mental arithmetic test at school because he could do it quicker and more accurately with his calculator. Another problem was his leaving tasks half done unless he had been told in detail precisely what was required. For example, when his mother said 'Can you run upstairs and see if I've left my library book on the bed?', Adrian answered 'Yes.' He went upstairs and saw the book, but left it where it was. He had

not taken on board that there was a second ambiguity in her words.

It is important that those who come into the autism spectrum, or have AS itself, should clearly understand their diagnosis. Parents, their well-meaning friends and loving grandparents often aid and abet each other in denying that there is anything unusual about the child. Denial and delay in recognizing the situation rob him of valuable time in which he could have been having appropriate treatment and learning how best to manage his particular problems. It is a relief to both child and parents alike when they know that the cause of his difference from other children is a subtle neurological variation in his brain.

It is often useful if teachers and friends are told about a child's AS, for then they will make allowances for his apparent gaucheness and inappropriateness – for instance, asking an elderly relative whether she is going to die yet. However, while you can talk about his AS in front of a very young child without any problem, to tell other people about it when he is older is playing fast and loose with his privacy and his pride. A parent may be thinking only of smoothing her child's path, but it is just as likely that he will be teased, imitated or bullied by the other children when they know. Or a high-profile crime by someone with a label of autism, well publicized by the media, can produce a wave of prejudice. It is impossible to un-say the diagnosis once it is out. So it needs thought and tact and you may have to choose whom to tell.

The variations of ASD, including AS, must be explained in a way that boosts rather than undermines the youngster's self-esteem. There are plenty of inspiring examples of AS. Think of Bill Gates of Microsoft, or Albert Einstein: outstanding achievers despite their developmental quirks, or Dr Temple Grandin and Liane Holliday Willey, two distinguished American women with AS, both of whom have written books on the subject.

There is nothing wrong or silly in concentrating on and enjoying 'doing one's own thing' – so long as other people are not bored beyond endurance by your talking about it. Similarly, with prefer-ring one's own company. In fact, many neurotypical adolescents are known for their social awkwardness and wanting to be alone, while a high proportion of AS teenagers want to have friends, including girl-or boyfriends, as well as having time on their own. There is nothing inherently wrong, either, in having a passion for sameness. Mark

Tully of the BBC has spoken of 'the solace of routine', something that we can all appreciate at times of stress.

> Our two adopted sons, Peter and Paul, have been with us since the ages of nine months and six weeks respectively. I was keen that they should know that they were adopted and that they should feel especially loved from day one. To this end, I sang them lullabies that brought in the word 'adopted' like a term of endearment, and as they grew older I told them stories in which 'adopted' doubled for words like 'good' or 'clever'. They tell me now, as adults, that they have always felt how special and wrapped in affection they are because of being adopted. The term 'Asperger' could be used in a similar way. Being different need not be a disadvantage.

Relationships with peers

Adolescence in AS ranges over a decade – years in which friendships are forged, careers and lifestyles planned, and adult independence shakily tried out. Sexual interest also develops slowly and hesitantly, but in AS youngsters dating may not start until the mid-twenties. Unlike other autistic individuals, adolescents with AS usually want to make relationships like neurotypicals of the same age, but they have very poor social and communication skills and imagination. Laughing at something sad is a commonplace. It is not a matter of lack of feeling, but of not knowing how to express it. Crying over something funny is more unusual.

To be accepted by his peers especially, an AS teenager must learn to modify tactless talk, in the form of unflattering – if true – personal remarks, and break the habit of interrupting and droning on and on about his own top interests. He must remember to continue being nice to someone by listening to him and paying compliments after he has already been accepted as a friend. He will need to practise putting himself in the other person's shoes; this is particularly difficult for him because of his lack of imagination. (See 'Making friends', in Chapter 11, for more on how to develop social skills.)

Acceptance by others and being attractive to them is helped by careful hygiene, grooming and gear – an area often overlooked by an AS boy or even a girl. The current teenage clothes and hairstyle, plus a smattering of 'in' words, are also useful if he is to fit in. A sense of humour also helps, especially laughing at other people's jokes. AS jokes are often a play on words that appeals to the intellect, but not to a sense of the ridiculous. They don't make you laugh aloud.

AS children share several problems with NT children:

- Stroppy behaviour.
- Moodiness.
- Depression.
- Social phobia.
- School refusal.
- Awkward, uncooperative behaviour – in a youngster with AS, this may be severe enough to be diagnosed as Oppositional Defiant Disorder (ODD). Its name describes the problem for parents, but at least it is clear-cut and cries out for ABA. Children with AS are notable for their excessive stubbornness, even on the most trivial-seeming matters, or any interruption to their rituals, so they can readily fall into ODD.

Kamran Nazeer
Kamran presented a different, less comprehensible, adolescent puzzle, ongoing into early adulthood, and has written a personal account entitled 'Learning to Talk', published in *Prospect*, April 2004. He did not begin to talk until he was two and a quarter, and later he only employed words for games he had invented. He recognized no other use for them since communication was irrelevant in his view. He approved of Isaac Newton's declining to meet the celebrities of the time, Voltaire and Benjamin Franklin. Kamran's behaviour was considered weird – for instance, spending the whole of break at school walking up and down the edge of the playground.

At the age of 12, around puberty, he was regarded as probably autistic, mainly because he so seldom spoke. He overheard his parents discussing this. He explained that he did not need friends because he had his thoughts, and he had no one to talk with. Kamran would answer a question and occasionally asked something factual, but he had no idea of how to turn this into a conversation, which anyway he had no wish for. This is not unusual in AS and other forms of ASD. When Kamran did speak, it was with extreme, but cold, unemotional politeness. Now and again he would say something appropriate and was considered a quiet, charming child.

As a teenager, his silence was felt to be strange and even menacing. Kamran believed his parents were afraid of him. It was at this stage that he could have fun with language, telling fantastic stories that were all lies. It then became clear that he had a remarkable intelligence, speaking three languages fluently, and easily winning a place at Cambridge. There the intellectual milieu suited him, and for the first time he made friendships. Today he has an encyclopaedic knowledge of world affairs and writes about philosophy, and enjoys juggling phrases to make them fit. A favourite quote of his is from Emerson: 'What you do speaks so loud, I cannot hear what you say.'

Because he is so well-read and intellectually sparkling, people often turn to Kamran for advice, but he admits that he does not relate to people on a feelings level, does not empathize, and cannot reassure them. He manages to live a successful life as a scholarly writer following a difficult adolescence and in spite of two handicaps: AS or High Functioning Autism (HFA), and giftedness. What a difficult time his parents must have suffered so far, despite their pride in him!

Any parent grappling with teenage AS problems must log on to the OASIS forum: Raising Teens and Young Adults (www.aspergersyndrome.org) for an account of what facilities are currently available for children of this age, especially in the USA.

Making friends with the opposite sex

One of the distinguishing features of people with AS is their wish and need to have relationships with other people, whereas those on other parts of the autistic spectrum may relate happily to inanimate objects or have an obsession with a particular body area in themselves or others. Like other teenagers, those with AS do develop new feelings of interest in the opposite sex, though usually more gently and gradually than in a so-called 'normal' or neurotypical person.

As adolescence is a protracted affair in AS, and because of their communication difficulties, teenagers with AS may lag behind their contemporaries, and miss out socially at the peak period for making lasting relationships, although they long to be accepted and have friends, including those of the opposite sex.

AS adolescents and young adults may include sexual behaviour among the ways they want to express themselves, but this is never the most important consideration. Personality traits rate higher than physical attributes with the AS youngster. Most appreciated are warm, extravert women who are strong and even inclined to be bossy – without undermining their partner's self-esteem. It is usually the girl who is the driving force, initiating the affair and keeping it on track.

Bertram

Bertram was attracted to girls in a typical AS fashion, using his brain to assess them. He was not turned on by their legs, breasts, bottoms or other erogenous areas, but looked for features that were not overtly sexual. Physical attraction was set off by their hair or eyes, but more often his feelings were kindled by the girl having interests he could share, intelligence he could measure and, most important of all, if she seemed to like him.

Bertram's thoughtful and affectionate relationship with Louise was built on his expertise with computers. She admired this and made him feel needed and wanted, a big plus point. He is now seriously considering marriage – in ten years' time, when they are 'more mature'. Louise may not want to wait, but Bertram has a one-track mind and has not considered her viewpoint.

Helping your teenager to communicate

What is obvious in the neurotypical world has to be learned and practised by an AS youngster – for instance, how to ask someone out. This involves remembering that it is the one who asks who is usually responsible for the bill!

Adolescent boys with AS, and to a lesser extent girls, need to be taught the social rules, including how to accept some rejections. In some cases they may benefit from social skills training (see Chapter 8). They are prone to do and say the wrong thing inadvertently because they often do not recognize and interpret the usual unspoken signals from others.

Another disadvantage is a tendency to speak too loudly which is embarrassing, or too quietly – both symptoms of nervousness, but irritating. Another mistake is constantly harping on about their special interest.

What can work really well is encouraging the youngster to look for a shared interest on which to base a relationship.

Adrian again

Adrian's father was a computer buff, clever and completely bound up in his subject. He was considered brilliant but eccentric: but at that time the autistic spectrum in adults was not well recognized. At 17, Adrian was a loner but he badly wanted a girlfriend – to be like the other boys. He was quiet and had no social skills – or friends. He seemed to prefer being on his own. Everyone said 'Adrian's just shy. He takes after his dad.' This was true, but no one considered AS. Fortunately for Adrian he was a good-looking fellow and a girl called Susan fell for him. She tentatively chatted him up and found they both enjoyed classical music. The effect of being liked, with the added bonus of a shared interest, set off Adrian's latent feelings.

For more on how to help your child to communicate, see Chapter 11.

Touch

A lot of AS adolescents are extremely sensitive to being touched, either by particular materials or by other people. It is difficult to say, however politely, 'I don't like being touched', but this is obviously better than visibly flinching.

Sex

It is particularly important that AS boys and girls are taught carefully and thoroughly, and well before puberty, about the practical and emotional aspects of intercourse, including contraception and sexually transmitted diseases (STD). They need to be especially warned about being exploited in this area, where they are unsophisticated in outlook and therefore vulnerable. The danger is even greater for girls with AS.

Some AS boys may have an innate distaste for physical intimacy or may prefer to delay it until a firm commitment has been proved, over several years. Indeed, 50 per cent of marriages involving a male partner with AS are never consummated. Others may desire closeness, but find it daunting. A quarter of young AS men would like to have more physical and sexual contact, as this can be a way of communicating feelings of love, which some AS males find easier than expressing themselves in words. This is in contrast to some autistic people, not of the Asperger type, who have not the slightest interest in sex and other personal relationships. Dustin Hoffman, in the film *Rain Man*, portrayed one such individual.

Couples

Despite the myth that people with AS cannot love, in fact they *do* love, marry and have children, though more AS men remain single. Once married, most men (75 per cent) remain faithful to their wives, compared with only around 5 per cent in the general public. Some AS men think that after the courting period, when they and their partner are committed, they no longer have to express loving and caring. One example of this was Robert, aged 22, who was amazed to learn from a counsellor that his wife felt neglected in these circumstances. 'But I told you last year that I loved you and I'd have let you know if that had changed,' he protested.

While some AS individuals will face sexual difficulties later on if they do decide to commit to a relationship, sympathetic and sensitive counselling can go a long way in overcoming these problems, and it may help some youngsters to be made aware now that help is available in this area if ever he or she should need it. The main difficulty an AS person can have is in reading the signals that should tell him what his partner wants from a relationship and engaging in loving sexual contact; and his difficulty in conveying his own needs and desires makes misunderstandings a constant danger. It is inspiring that love so often saves the day.

7
Co-existing conditions

AS is made up of variations in the development of the nervous system, and so presents a different picture with each individual. In one AS child there may be problems with language, in another an inability to play with toys, and in yet another a difficulty in relating to others. With such vague and variable boundaries it is not surprising that there is often an overlap with other problems, sometimes known as *co-morbid* conditions – in other words, disorders that frequently occur in association with Asperger Syndrome. What these conditions have in common is the underlying Pervasive Developmental Disorder (PDD) (see page vii).

Attention Deficit (AD)/Hyperactivity Disorder (HD)

This is the most common of the co-morbid conditions (*co* means 'with', *morbid* means 'to do with an illness or disorder') and is often regarded as part of AS. It comprises two groups of symptoms. One concerns difficulty in concentrating, paying attention, focusing on a particular subject and remembering it, while the other comprises non-stop restlessness and impulsivity to the point of recklessness. The child is constantly on the move, running, climbing and interfering with everything in sight. He cannot sit still in a chair for two minutes, let alone five. About 1.7 per cent of boys at primary school in the UK are judged to have AD/HD – and a quarter of that number of girls. The American figures are similar.

Robert
Robert was diagnosed with Attention Deficit Disorder (ADD) when he was six and at primary school. His inattention had come on some 18 months earlier, but it was assumed that he would get better when he started school. He didn't. At school his attention deficit was more obvious and he never seemed to take in the simplest lessons. His attention wandered and he would slip into a daydream in the middle of a meal, or get up and walk around. He would fully intend to do what the teacher said, but would forget what it was immediately. He was often in trouble over the things he did not do, but it always came as a surprise to him. Robert's

satchel was a jumble of chaos without any hint of organization, while another boy with ADD reacted the opposite way. He was obsessively tidy, becoming angry if anyone so much as touched one of his row of pencils, but he still lacked the ability to pay attention.

Robert was not overactive, but most children with serious attention problems have the full syndrome of AD/HD. Hyperactivity is far more disruptive than attention deficit and there is a constant risk of the child running into danger – literally. The parents can never relax and become exhausted, and some nursery or primary schools feel unable to cope with these children.

It has been claimed by some people that AD/HD is not a developmental disorder, but just 'children being children'. They only need to spend an afternoon looking after a hyperactive youngster to be disabused of this idea! Also, there is a genetic factor that accounts for AD/HD running in families. Some lively toddlers are overactive and can cause problems as soon as they can walk.

Drugs and the management of AD/HD

Jonathan

Jonathan's AD/HD came on when he was seven, but he had been a very restless baby and always into mischief as a toddler. He became impulsive and often disobedient, mainly because he had not listened – or remembered – what he had been told. As he was so difficult to manage, his mother asked the doctor if there was any treatment that would calm him down a little. The doctor sent him to a specialist with experience of AD/HD who said that a course of behavioural therapy would be the best option. The results were disappointing as Jonathan only followed the instructions while the therapist was there. Jonathan's mother was desperate and, rather against her principles, she agreed to a trial of medication. This was the nervous stimulant Ritalin (methylphenidate) – the last type of drug you would expect to help a hyperactive child. Paradoxically, in 40 per cent of cases it is the stimulant medicines that are effective in calming down the symptoms. Among these drugs, Ritalin has the fewest side-effects. It worked for Jonathan, but he had to continue taking it for nearly eight months before his symptoms came under control.

It is better to avoid using drugs on young children unless a thorough trial of the 'talking therapies' has proved ineffective. Fortunately, in most cases, as the youngster gets older the symptoms of AD/HD diminish and are generally gone by the time he reaches puberty. While the symptoms of AD/HD are in full spate, the child may be considered to have learning difficulties, but his intelligence shines through when these symptoms subside.

Parents can help at all stages – for instance, by making instructions uncomplicated and very specific, and reminding the youngster about them several times. Writing them down is more effective than just saying them. To help with focusing – for instance, on homework – it is important to remove all distractions and give rewards for tasks efficiently completed. Most AS children like diaries, notebooks, maps and diagrams and these all underpin concentration and memory.

Very recent research into AD/HD indicates that as well as the genetic element there is 'dysmaturity', a failure of the brain to develop fully. The part of the brain involved is the frontal lobe, one of the last parts to grow up. It may not become fully mature until well into adult life, and significantly it is concerned with personality and impulsivity. AD/HD may persist from childhood into adult life as an antisocial personality disorder or psychopathy. Some psychopaths are highly intelligent despite their poorly controlled impulses. This is concordant with the link with AS.

Collaboration between the specialist, who may be a psychiatrist, a psychologist or an educationist, and the parents and the patient is essential for this most troubling of disorders.

New research has also contributed to the management of a child or adult with AD/HD with the introduction of an effective medicine that is not a stimulant, and therefore safer. Its chemical or generic name is atomoxetine, and its trade name is Strattera (see page 76).

Anxiety states

We all experience anxiety at times, but in AS the general level of anxiety is higher than usual. Because the AS person's brain works differently, he has far fewer reliable expectations of others. The unpredictability of people is a constant source of anxiety to an AS child, who only longs for the security of sameness in his life.

Anxiety can set off several reactions which may be considered an integral part of AS:

1 Insomnia, especially difficulty in getting off to sleep, frequent waking in the small hours, and waking up unrefreshed.

2 Disturbed appetite: food can seem inedibly stodgy and tasteless even if it is lemon meringue pie; or, conversely, there is a compulsion to stuff food in all the time, especially sweets.
3 Tense, snappy mood, running into angry outbursts or tearfulness.
4 Extreme sensitivity. As we have seen, AS youngsters are often very sensitive to stimulation of the senses: sounds, lights, smells and, most of all, touch. The sensations can amount to pain. Anxiety sharpens these unpleasant sensory impressions and so, in a vicious circle, increases the anxiety.

A crisis can easily develop in these circumstances.

Specific causes for anxiety include changes at school, moving house or going on holiday, loss of a pet, crowds (or even being with two or three new people), and an illness or pain (although some AS youngsters have a high tolerance of pain).

Mothers can help by recognizing that difficult behaviour is very often a result of anxiety, and it is important for them to remain calm and loving and ask specifically about possible reasons for anxiety. Then they should stick to a routine, giving advance information of any deviation – even a treat event.

Depression

This is one of the most frequent co-morbid conditions, and while it is particularly likely to crop up with the hormonal upheavals of adolescence, those with AS may experience it at any time. Like anxiety, it can arise in reaction to a loss or trauma, but more often it develops for no clear reason. It is accompanied by a change in brain chemistry.

The American Academy of Child and Adolescent Psychiatry is concerned about the amount of 'hidden' depression and suffering among youngsters. It suggests a list of clues to watch out for:

- Headache or tummy ache.
- Poor sleep: particularly, early waking in a black mood.
- Change of appetite.
- Weight loss.
- Loss of interest in normal activities.
- Lack of energy.
- Irritability.
- Feelings of helplessness, hopelessness and guilt without cause.
- Slow-down of thinking and movement, and even movement of the bowels.

Bipolar disorder is an alternating state of depression and frenetic activity, interrupting other people and generally interfering. It runs in families, often starting in puberty.

In adults, two classes of antidepressants may help: the tricyclics such as amitriptyline, and the serotonin re-uptake inhibitors such as Prozac. These drugs are not suitable for adolescents or children, who may suffer severe, suicidal side-effects. Cognitive Behaviour Therapy (CBT), a talking treatment, is safe and generally successful at all ages. It is a training in positive thinking.

For a mild dip in spirits rather than clinical depression, an understanding discussion and praise of his good points lightens the youngster's mood. In AS children the virtues of honesty and truth stand out, as do the efforts they make to cope in a confusing world. Familiar activities and reinforcement of the affection that surrounds and protects them will act like a healing balm.

Obsessive Compulsive Disorder (OCD)

This affects one in 50 people, and frequently occurs in those with AS. For girls in particular it is often the first diagnosis, before the AS itself is recognized.

Obsessional thinking and incessant talking about one special subject is characteristic. Perfectionism is another facet of OCD, leading to compulsive rituals. These can involve food, which may have to be eaten in a certain order, or an idiosyncratic routine for dressing and undressing. The youngster is stubborn and dogmatic about his views and gets angry if he is thwarted. He may go on repeating something endlessly, trying to get it perfect. This is particularly irritating if it happens to be a piece of music.

Perfectionism can also make a child appear to be a bad sport because he cannot accept not being the winner in a game, and may refuse to go on playing if it looks as though he may lose. OCD is always accompanied by anxiety, and sometimes by depression. Treatment of the latter with medication or psychotherapy may greatly improve the OCD symptoms at the same time. The parents of 5–7 per cent of children with OCD also have the condition, indicating a definite genetic linkage.

Tourette's syndrome

This occurs in 1 in 2,000 children, with more than three-quarters of them being boys. It always begins before the age of 16, and is ten times more common in children than in adults. Its symptoms overlap with those of OCD, but the most characteristic feature is of multiple tics. These are sudden involuntary muscular twitches and more complex movements, and there is also a vocal type. This includes grunts and snarls and shouts. In a few cases it may consist of a string of obscenities, or just the odd swear word. There is hyperactivity, reminiscent of AD/HD, in the established disorder. The syndrome runs in families, indicating a genetic basis. Treatment with a major tranquillizer, haloperidol, reduces the symptoms in a substantial number of cases.

Phobias

Phobias are made up of episodes of extreme fear and panic. The sexes are affected equally. Childhood phobias are usually about animals, insects, the dark, school or death. They usually develop before the age of five, quite suddenly, and subside gradually from around the age of 11. In some cases, instead of a lessening of the symptoms, they become more severe after puberty and continue into adult life. More often, the phobias start in the teenage period and are at their worst between 17 and 30, when youngsters are at their most sensitive.

Social phobia

This is a fear of meeting strangers, speaking in public, eating in restaurants, or any situation where the victim feels exposed to other people's critical eyes. Just anticipating a party or some other social event is enough to set off the physical symptoms of acute anxiety: hot, scarlet blushing extending from the face down to the neck and chest, sweating and trembling, and a thumping heart.

Cognitive Behaviour Therapy (CBT), focusing on gradually facing the frightening situation, is the most effective treatment. It may take up to three months to work. Anxiolytic drugs such as Valium (diazepam) provide a quick fix, but are effective only temporarily. They act like a trap. Their effect is magical to start with, but larger and larger doses are needed and the victim becomes hooked on them.

Barbara

Barbara was 16 when she won a form prize; this involved walking up on to the platform on Speech Day to receive it. She became more and more anxious as she thought about this public ordeal. All the parents, staff and pupils would be there – suppose she stumbled, or dropped the prize just as Lady X, a local dignitary, was handing it to her? Barbara's feelings of anxiety culminated in a phobic attack – and then further phobic attacks.

The doctor prescribed a benzodiazepine anxiolytic drug, which suppressed the symptoms like magic, but left Barbara needing increasing amounts of the tablets. Her doctor then referred her to a clinical psychologist for a course of Cognitive Behaviour Therapy, which gradually exposed her to increasingly tense situations. This way, she learned to live through the phobic attacks, and in time she suffered fewer and fewer such attacks.

Barbara also had to contend with the added stresses of AS and being a teenager. Combined, these resulted in her having very poor social skills. A course of social skills training was a valuable source of increasing her confidence in dealing with other people and getting on with them. It involved learning the body language and practising exactly what to say in common social situations. These included greeting a friend, opening a conversation and, equally important, closing it on the right note. How to pay a compliment was another useful lesson. As her social confidence grew, she began to make a few friends.

Seizures

True epileptic seizures (fits) are caused by an electrical discharge in the brain. This is caused by genetic influences in 75 per cent of cases, and the remainder result from specific brain damage before or during birth. The essence of an epileptic seizure is a brief loss of consciousness, perhaps staring briefly into space, or sometimes falling down with jerking of the limbs, often with incontinence or tongue-biting. Anticonvulsant medication, under the guidance of a neurologist, usually controls the tendency to seizures satisfactorily. The disorder usually improves in young adulthood.

Apart from the inconvenience of suffering seizures, the main problems are social: the way epilepsy is regarded at school or work, or when contemplating getting married. Slowly this is changing as epilepsy comes out of the shadows. There are numerous other reasons than epilepsy for suffering seizures – some physical, some psychological. Physical causes include:

- A simple faint, caused by a drop in blood pressure as a result of shock or excessive heat.

- Hypoglycaemia: a low sugar level in the blood.
- Migraine.

Psychological and emotional causes include:

- Temper tantrums and breath-holding attacks (can occur in both AS children and other young children).
- Anger with aggressive outbursts, also in AS and other youngsters.
- Hyperventilation, over-breathing.
- Panic attacks.
- Night terrors.

Epilepsy and other types of seizure are relatively frequent in people with AS, and both involve an upset in the brain. An electroencephalogram (EEG) identifies genuine epilepsy.

Giftedness

You would not expect having exceptional intellectual gifts to be included as one of the co-morbid conditions that can cause problems for AS children. In fact, it can be almost as much of a handicap as subnormality. Anything that makes a child stand out, including being extra clever, makes him a target for bullying.

It used to be thought that all autistic children were especially gifted, and the same myth was applied all over again with reference to AS.

Some studies, by contrast, have indicated that 50 per cent of autistic children score as mentally retarded. Since some of these have responded so well to courses of ABA (Applied Behavioural Analysis), with some youngsters gaining as much as 20 per cent in IQ points, it casts doubt on the validity of the original testing. Although there may not be as many of the children with low IQs as had been thought, the number of highly gifted children with AS is still only a minority. It is rare for intellectual brilliance to extend across the board. It is characteristically patchy.

Simon

Simon was a maths phenomenon, working out fractions and long division at the age of three, and passing his university entrance examination at 11. On the other hand, he was no good at holding a knife and fork or catching a ball. Adults were impressed with Simon's facility with numbers, but condemned his difficulties – for instance, tying a shoelace – as a matter of laziness and generally poor co-operation. The only friends that he had used him to provide the answers to their homework, but never asked him to join in their games.

Simon's wholehearted fascination with maths problems, his pleasure in lying in bed thinking up new ones, and his endless, one-track talk made him a school bore. Sometimes, when he could not see a way of solving a particular puzzle, he would throw a tantrum in frustration. His teachers alternated between delight at his talents and irritation at his Asperger symptoms, including clumsiness and tactlessness. As he grew older, and after a long stint of ABA, Simon's social skills improved. With his maths expertise, he had an entrée to the normal academic world and he looks all set for a satisfying career.

8

Options and interventions

No intervention, ploy, treatment or training is the best one, or works for everyone. There is no magic bullet or simple quick-fix with medical, talking or behavioural management, although any of these may make a modest contribution either to suppressing the symptoms or enabling the youngster to cope with his AS and the anxiety that is bound to plague him some of the time.

The trick is to keep an open mind, cautiously trying out different methods, preferably on an AS parent's or teacher's recommendation, but not allowing yourself to be carried away by hope or by willing it to succeed. If a thorough trial produces no results, it is time to try another avenue – and meanwhile to revert to what comes naturally: loving your child and following his lead. There is a wide choice of alternative interventions and different children react differently to each one.

Behavioural treatments impinge directly on such symptoms as outbursts of anger, *perseveration* – that is, repeating the same words or actions over and over again – or the most common and fundamental of them all: a failure to communicate with other people and interact with them comfortably.

Social skills training

Poor or absent social skills are the bugbear of AS and HFA (High Functioning Autism) and affect some co-morbid disorders such as AD/HD or OCD (Obsessive Compulsive Disorder). Whatever else is needed, every AS youngster needs a course of social skills training, with follow-up along the same lines – indefinitely. This is essential if he is to be accepted by others of a similar age, escape a certain amount of the routine teasing dished out to anyone new, and achieve a degree of self-confidence.

Social skills are a must from nursery school through to secondary school, college and, finally, the wide world of employment and adult friends and partnerships. A key element is learning to be adaptable, a hurdle for sameness-loving AS children. An ABA programme (see below) can help, with practice in responding positively to changes in place, person or activity – for instance, a new classroom, a new teacher or a new game.

There are three ways of learning social skills:

1 By mixing in a group of five or six children, including AS, HFA or neurotypicals. (Those whose main disability is learning difficulty do not gel effectively.)
2 CBT (Cognitive Behaviour Therapy); see page 72.
3 ABA (Applied Behavioural Analysis); see page 69.

The essentials include:

• *Learning* how to respond to common social situations. This requires the exact words to be used and rehearsed.
• *Practice*, preferably with other children by role-playing.

For more on learning to master social skills, see the advice in Chapter 11 on Lifestyle.

Occupational therapy

Most of us know someone, neurotypical or otherwise, who benefited from being taught, and practising, everyday skills after an illness or because of some other handicap.

Apart from such basics as washing, tooth-cleaning, dressing and grooming, occupational therapy can also apply to running, skipping, hopping, throwing and catching a ball, modelling, writing and drawing – simple skills that AS children may find very difficult. One of the reasons is their often extreme sensitivity, affecting any of the senses. This is Sensory Integration Disorder (SID). Between 12 and 20 per cent of all children, especially those with AS, have some degree of this, and 80 per cent of them are boys. It can be the cause of AS babies flinching from such contact as hugging and kissing.

While extra sensitivity to touch is the most frequent problem in AS, other senses may also be affected: smell, sight, taste, balance or hearing. The tiniest sensory stimulus can cause discomfort and distress, to the level of panic or actual pain. The child's natural reaction is to avoid it, but when that is not possible to scream or have a tantrum. Small children with AS are often blamed, unfairly, for lacking normal, warm, loving feelings, even for their mothers, because they flinch or cry or shut down all reaction temporarily at the most loving touch.

Billy, aged four, screamed when his Aunty Rose gave him a

gentle cuddle, but when he had an injection at the doctor's he did not even flinch. Also, Billy and his cat, named Cat, enjoyed rolling on the floor together.

Sensory experience is the way babies and children learn about the world and the meaning of what they feel – for instance, the sound that means a piano or a robin, the brightness that means sunshine or a candle, and a vast range of subtly different sensations all connected with emotions. It was Dr A. Jean Ayres, around 50 years ago, who coined the phrase *sensory integration* for this link between sensation, meaning and feelings. It arises through the development of the nervous system, and in children with Pervasive Developmental Disorder (PDD) faults in sensory integration are common. This leads to the condition Sensory Integration Disorder (SID). Dr Ayres strongly believed that the child's brain could be retrained to correct SID. ASD and AS itself are forms of PDD.

Sensations come from the skin and mouth, the balance organ in the ear, the taste buds, chemical receptors in the nose, and the muscles and joints which provide ongoing information about the body's movements and posture. Some AS children with SID have a strange running action, strike odd poses, and appear clumsy and awkward. Their co-ordination is faulty, which makes them hopeless at school games.

Although quite a few AS youngsters are super-sensitive to touch, sound, bright lights, smell or taste, others have blunted sensations so that they do not feel pain when other people would. *Synaesthesia* is a mixture of the senses. Bob, for instance, always saw sounds as different colours. Some neurotypical people have this interesting experience for no apparent reason, or they can bring it on by such drugs as LSD. AS children quite often get their sensations mixed up due to a fault in their sensory integration.

Luke Jackson's younger brother, also an Aspie, claps his hands over his ears when a light is switched on. He used to have skin sensitivity and hated the feeling of his clothes touching him, so he often took them off. Then he discovered that wearing them inside out was a help, especially if they were green.

Sensory Integration Training (SIT)

The treatment for SID is based on stimulating the sensation that is causing problems for the youngster, so that he learns to recognize it and can be helped to interpret it correctly, and adjusting the strength and character of what he feels – say, a tickle, a scratch or a blow. A skilled therapist is required to guide a child through a course of Sensory Integration Training (SIT). Improvement can be expected over the next few weeks. Occupational Therapy at the same time is often helpful.

Auditory Integration Training (AIT)

There is a special name for the disorder associated with faults in auditory (hearing) integration: Central Auditory Processing Disorder (CAPD). In this case, the child hears sounds normally, but is unable to make proper sense of them. Children with this problem, including some with AS, have hyperacute hearing, and some everyday sounds set off an extreme reaction – pain or panic, irrational anger or an emotional switch-off. They also have a difficulty with focusing their attention on listening.

Sound sensitivity affects 40 per cent of all types of autistic children, and up to 75 per cent of those with AS have some degree of it. The worst sounds are:

• Sudden loud noises.
• Screaming crowds.
• Sirens and alarms.
• High-pitched whistles.
• A crying baby.
• Some high-pitched voices.

Auditory Integration Therapy (AIT) comes in several versions, all based on listening programmes. Two Frenchmen, working separately, founded the first of these in the 1960s. Dr Alfred Tomatis developed his audio-psycho-phonology on a basis of 100 hours of listening to high-frequency sounds including familiar voices, songs, stories and music. Dr Guy Berard rubbished this method and promoted the idea that 'hearing equals behaviour'. His timetable ran on half-hour listening slots, separated by at least three hours, over a period of ten days. High and low frequencies were eliminated. Guidance and supervision by an audiologist is necessary if either of these methods is used, and they are expensive.

Several other programmes are available at a much lower cost on a CD-ROM – for instance, Earobics, Train Time and Fast For Word. The aim in all these is to marry the hearing experience with meaning. Parents can help via patience and understanding, as always, and avoiding situations such as crowds where the upsetting noises are likely to occur. They should not talk over the sound of TV or radio, but should get the youngster's full attention before speaking and then use short, simple sentences. Children with CAPD should be taught to ask for explanations and repeats of things they do not understand.

Applied Behavioural Analysis (ABA)

Sometimes known as Lovaas treatment after Dr O. Ivar Lovaas, one of the early workers in the field, Applied Behavioural Analysis (ABA) is one of the most successful interventions. It is a scientific approach to reducing unwanted behaviour, and finally eliminating it, while at the same time teaching and fostering good social relations and some self-help skills in a structured learning programme. ABA was introduced in the 1960s in Los Angeles, with the aim of teaching and helping autistic children to behave like 'normal' or neurotypical youngsters. It is best begun in early childhood, but is also of value in adults of all ages, including some 50-year-olds. It is particularly effective when the symptoms have 'come out of nowhere' or 'make no sense'. The underlying theory of ABA, enunciated by psychologist Dr Bobby Newman, states that all behaviour follows certain laws. These can be described in an ABC format. A is the antecedent – that is, what it was that led to the target behaviour in the first place. B is the actual behaviour, and C is its consequence – that is, what happens as a result, whether or not this was what was intended.

Joe
Joe found maths problems confusing and had developed a habit of humming loudly and tunelessly whenever they were given as an exercise in class, making it difficult for the other children to concentrate. Joe's teacher said that if he did not stop it he must stay in at break. She had hoped to discourage Joe's humming, but in the event it became worse. The punishment acted paradoxically as a *reinforcer* since being kept in saved Joe from having to go out in the playground where he was often teased.

Analysis: the antecedent situation was the maths test, the relevant

69

behaviour was Joe's humming, and the consequence had turned out to be a reinforcer.

The object of ABA treatment is to discourage unwanted or antisocial behaviour and reward or reinforce socially acceptable actions or speech, and self-help skills that most other people take for granted – like greeting friends or apologizing if you accidentally step on their toes. It is useful to build up a small treasury of useful social phrases (see page 97). When ABA was first introduced there was definite punishment for undesirable behaviour, but this has now been dropped in favour of rewards for doing what is desirable and ignoring 'bad' behaviour. The therapist is meant to speak in a neutral tone, unless he is deliberately using praise as a reward, but some children find this unpleasant, even threatening. For ABA to be effective, parents, teachers, grandparents and others who are concerned with the Aspie child must co-operate in applying a response they have all agreed upon whenever one of the target behaviours, desirable or otherwise, occurs.

Gareth again
Gareth was told, by whichever adult might be present, to put his hand over his mouth every time he had an impulse to scream, delaying it at first for one minute, then, two, progressively. Every success was met with a reward that might be lavish praise, a biscuit, a hug or a tickle, or choosing a bedtime story. The learning process advanced in small, easily achieved steps, each one repeated whenever necessary. When Gareth had gained reasonable control of his screaming, the approved response would be allowed to fade.

In 1987 Lovaas published a study on 19 children with autistic disorders who received 40 hours a week of one-to-one therapy using his method. There was a remarkable increase in the youngsters' IQ, averaging 20 points, and nine children (47 per cent) passed the first year at a standard primary school. Eight of these, when they were all re-examined in 1993, had lost none of their recently learned skills. By this time, they were 13.

What a child gains by the ABA system encompasses a vital facet of learning: the principle of small steps. Goals and rewards make everything into a minor triumph, a boost to the youngster's confidence and self-esteem. These are often sadly lacking in AS. A trained, certified therapist is needed to run a course of ABA, but these are in short supply and there may be a two-year waiting list in some areas.

Doing it yourself

The alternative is for the parents to become the therapists. Most parents of AS children are both bright and devoted, and they can read up and apply the necessary techniques for most treatments – but ABA is particularly tricky.

However, there is the problem of burn-out. Treatment can take as much as six hours a day, which may be impractical for many busy parents. Added to this difficulty is the possibility of psychological fatigue in both parent and child, especially if several training courses are running at the same time – for instance, a social skills group and speech therapy. A mother may find herself criticizing the treatment and feeling pessimistic about this and her own parenting, while the youngster reacts by becoming less co-operative. It is then time for a therapy holiday for a few weeks, and a gentle start-up to follow.

'Extinction burst' is another difficulty. This is similar in its cause to burn-out, but specific to ABA. In other words, concentrated ABA can lead to an actual increase in the frequency and severity of the unwanted behaviour that was being targeted.

Keith

Keith's problem was his poor attention, his inability to remain in his chair in class, and his tendency to daydream when he was sitting down, and to forget whatever he had just been told. Information or instructions had to be given in bite-size chunks, clearly and specifically, and Keith had to repeat each one of them immediately, either verbally or in writing. This backed up the ABA that was helping him to sit in his place for increasing periods until he could manage a whole lesson.

It was important to keep detailed notes on each session to give a check on progress or lack of it, and in the latter case to backtrack over the events leading up to it. Occasionally there is a breakthrough after the first or second session of ABA, but usually it is a matter of a series of small improvements. Extinction burst meant that Keith became extremely restless – even disruptive – in class, after a concentrated period of ABA. Fortunately, the 'burst' is usually temporary, briefly preceding the final elimination of the unwanted behaviour.

Cognitive Behaviour Therapy (CBT)

This treatment, poached from straight psychiatric practice, assumes that all psychological disorders have both cognitive (thinking) and behavioural (doing) components. For example, repetitive morbid thoughts precede behaviour such as self-harm in severe depression. In obsessional disorders, such as often occur in AS, unbidden repetitive thoughts go hand in hand with repetitive rituals. CBT uses a dual approach. In the cognitive part the therapist aims at changing faulty thinking – for example, correcting irrational fears. The behavioural element in this case would be to work up in small steps to doing the very thing the sufferer is afraid of – for instance, entering a crowded room.

Unlike the reward system of ABA, CBT relies on logical argument. This is especially acceptable to older children with AS, whose powers of reasoning are well developed. Christopher, the fictional hero of Mark Haddon's famous novel, portrays brilliantly the AS characteristic of logical but concrete or literal thinking.

Bridget

Bridget was 14 when she found herself friendless and unhappy, and unable to mix with her own age group. She had mild AS or HFA (High Functioning Autism) and had got through her early years with no other help but the support of sympathetic parents and a first teacher who had experience of children with AS. In adolescence, Bridget began to stand out as different. She kept up well with her schoolwork but, unlike other teenagers, especially the girls, she showed no interest in her appearance. Clothes seemed irrelevant to Bridget and she looked slovenly and grubby, changing neither her underwear nor top clothes unless her mother reminded her.

Bridget's personal hygiene was no better, and she did not bother to clean her teeth regularly or comb her hair before she went out. To make matters worse, since she did not have the social skills to mix with her peers, she did not pick up teen language, tastes in music or interest in football. Yet like the other children of her age, she wanted to have friends. Her mother tried to find a teenage group for her. There was nothing local, but she did find an excellent, all-purpose online group on Raising Teens and Young Adults, accessed through the OASIS website (www.aspergersyndrome.org.). Another good source of help was the book by Brenda Smith Myles and Diana Adreon: *Asperger Syndrome and Adolescence: Practical Solutions for School Success.*

ABA might have benefited Bridget, but her high IQ made CBT ideal for her. In Bridget's case, her mother saved the day. At an alumni get-together she sought out all the mothers who had been at school with her and found several with daughters of the same age as Bridget, but without AS. Encouraged by their mothers, two girls arranged to help Bridget learn the ropes of modern adolescent living, and became her friends. The social aspects of a group or, in Bridget's case, her two friends, helped her behaviour to become more acceptable among her peers during this key period in her life. The real saviours, as in so many cases, were her parents.

The parents of Asperger children stand out as among the most devoted and enterprising of a wonderful bunch of human beings.

Speech and language therapy

This is essential for the majority of AS children who are likely to have speech and language disabilities. The following are clues that the therapy is needed:

- Misinterpretation of other people's words and actions.
- Cannot understand non-verbal communication, e.g. smiles, gestures.
- Often uses and interprets language literally.
- Odd way of speaking, maybe monotonous.
- Difficulty in opening or closing a conversation gracefully.
- Often misses the point, but remembers the detail precisely.
- Unaware of the other person's reaction, e.g. boredom or hurt feelings.
- Difficulty in dealing with abstract concepts such as time or ideas.
- Slow to answer questions or otherwise respond in conversation.

Speech and language therapy is an educational specialty especially useful in ASD, and helpful in social learning. Parents can help on the homework front – as directed.

Social stories and comic strips

If you can draw matchstick men you can illustrate words, stories and conversations and everyday activities: a great help in explaining these to AS youngsters. It is also a way of getting some insight into what the speaker may be thinking, in a bubble. For instance, if a teacher says 'Pull your socks up' he means 'Try harder', or when he says 'Pay attention', it doesn't mean you have to give him any money, but only to listen carefully.

9

Medication

There is no magic pill that will cure AS, although the drug companies are constantly bringing out new products. Chemicals cannot change the genes, nor erase the effects of little variations in development or minor degrees of brain damage that may occur in the womb. These are the underlying causes of AS. Medicines may modify some of the symptoms, but are most effective with the co-morbid disorders that often accompany it. These include:

- AD/HD.
- Anxiety states.
- Depression.
- Bipolar affective disorder.
- Obsessive Compulsive Disorder (OCD).
- Social and other phobias.
- Tourette's syndrome.
- Fits.
- Insomnia.

AD/HD is a prime example. The characteristic hyperactivity and impulsivity, and the less obtrusive inattention, are all reduced, paradoxically, by some stimulant drugs. It takes a period of four to eight weeks.

Some people have an almost superstitious distrust of all drugs, but there is no doubt about their efficacy in this devastating disorder. The stimulant most often employed is methylphenidate (trade names Ritalin, Concerta XL, Tranquilyn). This has fewer unwanted side-effects than the others, and has been in use since 1955. None of the stimulants should be given to children under the age of six; or those weighing less than 70 kg; nor to anyone with high blood pressure; a family history of tics or Tourette's syndrome; or if they are taking an antidepressant, especially an MAOI (see below), or a few less of the less common medicines, or alcohol.

In all cases, a thorough trial of psychological or behavioural treatment should be carried out first – for example, CBT, ABA or simple, supportive psychotherapy. This may not work on its own; likewise, the medication may not be effective unless it is accompanied by ongoing behavioural modification.

Stimulant medication

- Methylphenidate (vs).
- Dexamphetamine (Dexedrine) and combinations of different amphetamines.
- Other amphetamines, e.g. methamphetamine (Desoxyn).
- Pemoline (Cylert).

These are all wake-up medicines, increasing alertness and sensitivity except in those with AD/HD who react in the opposite way.

Dosage for methylphenidate

Children over 6 and up to 10 (not adults), 5 mg once or twice daily, increasing as needed by 5 mg weekly to a maximum of 60 mg daily.

Possible side-effects of methylphenidate

Include: anxiety, loss of appetite and weight loss, insomnia and palpitations, irregular periods and an uneasy lethargy. Methylphenidate has the fewest side-effects among the stimulants, and is best known under the trade name of Ritalin.

Amphetamines have the serious disadvantages of tolerance and dependence. They lose their efficacy over time and require increasing doses, with the risk of addiction. However, amphetamines are less likely than methylphenidate to trigger an increase in seizure frequency in a child with epilepsy. In some children, a tendency to tics and Tourette's syndrome is enhanced, but not caused, by stimulants and an occasional major unwanted effect of stimulant treatment is an increase instead of a reduction in the original symptoms of AD/HD in some children.

Breakthrough: atomoxetine

In 2004, the first non-stimulant treatment for AD/HD was introduced: atomoxetine (Strattera). It acts against the symptoms as well as methylphenidate or dexamphetamine, but without the risks of taking a stimulant – including the addictive potential of the amphetamines. Atomoxetine reaches its full effect in six to nine weeks, and a single 40 mg dose remains active for 24 hours, so one daily dose is sufficient for children and adolescents. It can also be given to young adults who may still have some of the symptoms. It is claimed that it also improves the social and general psychological state of the patient. It does not increase the likelihood of tics or the other symptoms of Tourette's syndrome.

MEDICATION

Dosage for atomoxetine

For adults and children who weigh over 70 kg, the dose is 40 mg daily for 7 days, then an increase to a regular 80 mg daily (maximum daily 100 mg). Younger, lighter children are given 0.5 mg per kg body weight for starters, increasing to a steady 1.2 mg per kg, but children younger than 6 are not admissible – as with the stimulant medicines.

Especially careful supervision is needed in cases with kidney or liver disease or blood pressure that is too high or too low. Atomoxetine interacts with MAOIs, the Prozac-type antidepressants and salbutamol.

Possible side-effects of atomoxetine

Include: reduced appetite with weight loss, insomnia *or* sleepiness, sore eyes, headache, stomach pain, or bed-wetting.

Norman

Norman was one of the 3.5 per cent of school-age children with AD/HD of the hyperactive type. His liveliness kept his parents and teacher so distracted that it was not until he had been taking atomoxetine for six months, and his symptoms had subsided, that his parents began to worry about his solitariness in school and his all-consuming passion for insects and their lifestyles. He was diagnosed with AS when he was eight, and linked into an Asperger social group.

Anxiolytics

Anxiety states occur frequently in children with AS, and especially in those who also have an extra (co-morbid) problem. The drugs that help are the anxiolytics. The most common ones are the *benzodiazepines*, famously diazepam, the trade name for Valium. Alprazolam (Xanax) is a short-acting preparation, lorazepam (Ativan) is intermediate, and chlordiazpoxide (Librium) is long-acting. They all work like a charm, and equally seductively. They rapidly and effectively banish the unpleasant physical symptoms like tremor, sweating, rapid heartbeat and indigestion, as well as the psychological tension and inability to concentrate. However, without a constant increase in dosage they lose their power, so they are extremely addictive. Currently, there is a worldwide increase in their use.

To make matters worse, it is difficult to get off these drugs, especially with higher doses and if they have been used for more than two or three weeks. Withdrawal must be gradual as there is a high risk of rebound, with the symptoms returning tenfold. They should never be given to children or those with AS, however anxious and distressed they are. They should also be avoided for everyone else, except in cases of severe, incapacitating anxiety in those over 18, when the maximum length of treatment should be a fortnight. The exception to the ban on benzodiazepines for children is occasionally lifted in the case of small doses of diazepam itself for a minimum period.

Non-benzodiazepine drugs are not as effective in treating anxiety, but incomparably safer. They include:

- Buspirone (Buspar) is chemically unique, effective in reducing anxiety within a week, and is not addictive.
- Propanolol (Inderal) and oxprenolol (Trasicor) are beta-blockers: they reduce tremor, palpitations and gastric upset, but not the mental side of anxiety.
- Antihistamines – for instance, hydroxyzine (Atarax).
- Venlafaxine (Efexor), a relaxing antidepressant.

None of these is recommended by the manufacturers for those under the age of 18.

Antidepressants

Depression often occurs in conjunction with anxiety or as a reaction to the stress of living with AS, particularly among teenagers struggling to come to terms with the realization that they are different from the usual run of youngsters. Unfortunately, while antidepressant drugs are often helpful and usually safe for depressed adults, in young people they can make the symptoms worse, even leading to suicidal attempts in a few adolescents. Extremely careful supervision is a must, especially with the newer, more effective preparations, the SSRIs (selective serotonin reuptake inhibitors).

These drugs are not generally recommended for children or adolescents. They also interact with the whole MAOI group of antidepressants, some neuroleptics and anti-epileptics, lithium and alcohol.

Types of tricyclic antidepressants (TCADs)

Tricyclic antidepressants (TCADs) are very long established. Their possible side-effects include dry mouth and blurred vision, constipation, racing pulse, low blood pressure and palpitations. More importantly, they can be dangerous in overdose or to people with a heart disorder. They too are not positively recommended in England, except in special cases such as bed-wetting (enuresis).

Sedating types of TCADs

- Amitriptyline (Elavil).
- Dosulepin (Prothiaden).
- Doxepin (Sinequan).
- Trimipramine (Surmontil).
- Lofepramine (Lomont, Gamanil).

Stimulating types of TCADs

- Imipramine (Tofranil).
- Clomipramine (Anafranil).
- Nortriptyline (Allegron), used for bed-wetters below the age of 6.

Neither of these types should be given within 14 days of taking an MAOI antidepressant, or 21 days in the case of clomipramine or imipramine. They interact badly with anti-epileptics, drugs to lower the blood pressure, and those for treating thyroid disorders.

MAOIs

Another family of antidepressants, the monoamine oxidase inhibitors (MAOIs), involves another neurotransmitter. They are sometimes successful when other types have failed, and can be helpful in OCD. Their big disadvantage is that they react dangerously, occasionally fatally, with certain foodstuffs. These foodstuffs are:

- Broad bean *pods*.
- Banana *skins*.
- Meat extracts (Bovril, Oxo).
- Yeast extract (Marmite, and other yeast extracts).
- Cheese, except cottage cheese.
- Chocolate.

- Vegetarian 'meats'.
- Food that has 'gone off'.
- Alcohol, especially wine and beer.

They also clash with narcotic analgesics (painkillers) such as pethidine; stimulants; buspirone (Buspar); carbamazepine (Tegretol); the tricyclic and SSRI antidepressants (they must not be taken within five weeks of a dose of Prozac, two weeks with others of the group).

Types of MAOI drugs

- Phenelzine (Nardil).
- Tranylcypromine (Parnate).
- Moclobamide (Manerix), also used for social phobia.

Atypical antidepressants

There are a handful of medicines that do not fit into any particular groups, but have proved themselves useful in some cases of depression:

- Trazodone (Molipaxin, Desyrel), useful for panics and disturbed sleep.
- Mirtazapine (Zispin, Soltab), also used for panic attacks.
- Nefazodone (Serzone), also given for panic disorder.
- Bupropion (Wellbutrin, Zyban), also used in AD/HD and smoking addiction.
- Maprotiline (Ludiomil).

Mood stabilizers

Bipolar illness, in which periods of severe depression alternate with weeks or more of over-cheerful liveliness and excitement, cannot be treated with antidepressants without leading to a manic state. There is one tailor-made preparation for this disconcerting disorder, lithium.

Lithium

Lithium salts, usually the carbonate (Priadel, Camcolit, Liskonum), level out the peaks and troughs of mood but not without a price. The level of lithium in the serum has to be maintained within a narrow range (0.5–0.8 mmols per litre), necessitating regular blood tests. Too low a level is useless, but too high is extremely dangerous. The symptoms of toxicity (poisoning) are vomiting, twitching, drowsiness, slurred speech and confusion. They demand urgent treatment in hospital.

Lithium interacts with water tablets (diuretics) and NSAIDs (nonsteroidal anti-inflammatory drugs) used widely in arthritis and other painful conditions, and also carbamazepine, phenytoin, haloperidol, metoclopramide and steroid medicines. It is not recommended under the age of 12, and even then only in cases of excessive mood swings, such as occur in some children with AS.

Lithium is also used in recurrent depression without the 'up' phase.

Carbamazepine (Tegretol)

This is an anti-epileptic which can be used as a mood stabilizer in children aged six and upwards; it has been in use since 1968. Others are:

- Lamotrigine (Lamictal).
- Phenytoin (Epanutin).
- Sodium valproate (Epilim).

Valium-type drugs are also used, especially to calm someone down in an excitable, hypomanic phase.

Antihypertensives

Antihypertensives are drugs that reduce the blood pressure. They are used in migraine and in AS children with hard-to-manage attacks of anger, agitation, impulsivity or self-harm, and also in Tourette's syndrome. Reducing the blood pressure has the opposite effect to anger or excitement, and was the object of our ancestors' use of bleeding and cupping for their restless, overwrought patients. Drugs used in this way are:

- Clonidine (Dixarit, Catapres).
- Propanolol (Inderal).

Neuroleptics

These are also known as antipsychotics or major tranquillizers. They are used in serious mental illness, particularly schizophrenia, and have a powerful calming effect. In low dosage they are used in Tourette's syndrome, tics and tantrums. The medication takes effect immediately and will cut short, to five minutes, a tantrum that might otherwise have gone on for half an hour. Neuroleptics act similarly against episodes of violence and other uncontrollable outbursts. In very small doses they are useful in anxiety states and in the frustration that upsets AS children who are misunderstood.

Unpleasant side-effects of these drugs, for instance muscle spasms, including the eye muscles, may come on soon after taking a few doses of the drug, but the worst type – tardive dyskinesia – does not arise until the drug has been used for many months. Involuntary mumbling movements of the mouth in particular may continue indefinitely. There is a risk of Parkinsonism from taking these drugs, which also involves a disorder of movement, and a small danger of an acute confusional state with a high temperature that is life-threatening, neuroleptic malignant syndrome.

Haloperidol (Haldol, Serenace) is the neuroleptic most frequently used in Tourette's syndrome. It is a well-established, 'typical' neuroleptic. These sorts are the most likely to cause side-effects. There is also a group of chemically different and varied 'atypical' neuroleptics, which are more effective and have fewer side-effects.

Typical neuroleptics

- Haloperidol (Haldol, Serenace).
- Trifluoperazine (Stelazine).
- Thioridazine (Melleril).
- Pimozide (Orap).
- Chlorpromazine (Largactil, Thorazine).

Atypical neuroleptics

- Clozapine (Clozaril).
- Risperidol (Risperdal), recommended in bipolar illness, from the age of 15 upwards.
- Aripiprazole (Abilify), the newest of them, and claimed to have fewer side-effects.

Hypnotics (sleeping pills)

Very occasionally a child or adult with AS should be given a sleeper, but the healthiest way to bring sleep to an overtired and restless or overexcited youngster who cannot settle is the labour-intensive human method. This can be singing to the very young; reading a story to the slightly older child; gentle, soothing talk with the theme of problems ironed out; a stroll through a stretch of beautiful country; or riding in a boat floating down the river.

Sleeping pills soon lose their efficacy if they are used regularly, so they should never be used for more than two or three days at a time, at any age, and preferably as a one-off.

My own preference is for my Granny's recipe: a warm, milky drink and a Rich Tea biscuit – nice but not addictive.

10

Miracle cures

Every now and again someone enthusiastically claims to have found a cure for AS. This new treatment seems to provide the perfect answer for one person at least. They convince others that it will work for them too, and something like a crusade can develop. After all, isn't this what all the parents, friends and teachers of children with AS dream of – a kind of magic: a particular drug or training programme that will banish the symptoms and problems of AS speedily and permanently?

Unfortunately, such a marvellous outcome is too good to be true for everyone. To start with, AS is not an illness that can be eradicated, but an inbuilt part of the person's constitution, based on his genes and minute variations in brain development in the womb. Both of these are permanent and unchangeable. Second, if all traces of AS could be erased or 'cured' – so would the child's personality. Literally, he would no longer be the same person. Another big stumbling block is that we do not know what causes AS, except that it is biological. Research into autism, and specifically AS, is going on all the time and the AS website is spattered with requests for volunteers to take part in new studies. The future is full of promise.

Critical evaluation is based on careful observation and testing, and sober statistics. Particularly where medication is involved, 'double blind' trials are essential – that is, testing the new 'cure' against the standard treatment, with neither the subject nor the doctor knowing which drug the person is taking.

The most recent of such 'cures' to be tried was the hormone secretin. This was launched with a fanfare of publicity, but a number of trials have shown it to be ineffective.

A lack of trace elements and vitamins in the diet – such as zinc, magnesium, calcium, DMG (dimethylglycine), or fish oils omega 3, 6 or 9 – has also been blamed for autism, but giving supplements of these has no effect on the key AS symptoms. Epsom salts put in the bath have also failed as a cure, despite keen backing for a short time. The same applies to the use of horse manure applied externally, which briefly aroused some interest, unlikely though it seems.

Diet

Far and away the most frequently tried ploys are special diets, usually cutting something out, especially the protein called casein in dairy products, and gluten from wheat. Egg products may be singled out as affecting others. Food sensitivity, including the allergic type involving the immune system, can have a general effect on health. Nowadays, while few people regard the GF/CF (gluten-free/casein-free) diet as an actual cure for autism, many AS children and their parents see it as improving their quality of life with greater openness and self-confidence. The avoidance of certain food additives is often practised with the diet. These additives include the sweeteners aspartame and saccharin; the preservatives sulphur dioxide, nitrates and sodium metabisulphite; the flavour enhancers monosodium glutamate and sodium inosinate; and the synthetic colourings tartrazine, brown FK and erythrosine. Luke Jackson, author of *Freaks, Geeks and Asperger Syndrome*, believes this restricted diet has 'changed the lives' of himself and his autistic brothers.

Food sensitivity affects 10 per cent of children, those under three in particular, but 20 per cent of adults report that certain foods disagree with them. Some food sensitivity is a type of allergy – that is, it involves the immune system. Peanut allergy is one of the most widespread. Brazils, almonds and hazelnuts have a similar effect. Other allergens are fish, especially shellfish, and infection with Candida and other yeasts acts in the same way.

Allergy is believed by some to trigger the symptoms of autism in the presence of an underlying tendency to the condition. Allergy induced Autism (A i A) is the name of a charity committed to the idea that allergy is at the root of autism. Treatment for allergy will certainly benefit the symptoms of allergy, but is not a cure for autism.

Neither restrictions nor food supplements have been shown to have any effect on the key features of AS: the triad of impairments – difficulty in interacting with other people; poor communication with them, both verbally and by body language; and lack of imagination, causing an inability to empathize. Also key is the characteristic passion for sameness, leading to a familiar, narrow, repetitive pattern of activities.

Vitamins and herbs

Although diet is the most talked about 'cure' for AS, a shortage of certain vitamins is constantly being reconsidered as a cause of ASD, including AS. In particular, the B group of vitamins are often in the spotlight since autistic children use a little more of these than other people.

Mega doses of Vitamin C, ascorbic acid, or Vitamin B6, pyridoxine, are sometimes recommended, but the latter can be dangerously toxic to the nervous system. High doses of Vitamin C are harmless, and slightly stimulating. As mentioned above, the trace elements and the minerals magnesium, zinc and calcium have also been tried, but although they may improve the diet, they have no effect on the core symptoms of AS.

Herbal remedies are used for everything, including AS, by herbalists and they can relieve some of the related symptoms. St John's Wort is useful for lifting depression and some of the herbal remedies can be used to relieve the anxiety that AS children are prone to develop. Harmless, non-addictive plant sedatives are invaluable for soothing emotional outbursts. Motherwort tea, containing also valerian, skullcap, mistletoe and balm, is said to 'restore calm and poise' quickly. Eating two or three bananas daily is also recommended.

Behavioural training and educational programmes

Behavioural training and educational programmes cannot alter structural differences in children's brains, but may modify the way their brains and emotions work.

Sensory Integration Therapy (SIT) and Auditory Integration Therapy (AIT)

As seen earlier, both of these have been hailed as cures for autism, but are now accepted as sometimes useful, but not exceptional, treatments. They have the disadvantage, which they share with educational programmes, of taking so many months, even years, to produce results that they are often abandoned as ineffective before that. Yet these probably provide as near a cure as any therapy. Dr Alfred Tomatis's audio-psycho-phonology and Dr Guy Berand's form of AIT are particularly beneficial for children with Central

Auditory Processing Disorder (CAPD), but do not amount to a cure (see page 68).

Speech and language programmes

While speech and language therapy helps many AS children (see Chapter 8), it will not produce a cure. This is also the case with programmes involving listening to music, either carefully chosen, or whatever is at hand; there seems little difference in the results. Some 40 per cent of AS children and adults have increased sound sensitivity, and up to 75 per cent show at least some signs of it. There are several sound programmes and Earobics is typical.

Facilitated communication was introduced with high expectations in the 1970s. It comprises one-to-one sessions in which the therapist helps the child to express himself by supporting his arm or a finger and moving it to emphasize his words and reveal their meaning. There is a sophisticated jargon that accompanies this. Exaggerated claims have been made for this treatment, but studies have shown them to be invalid.

Educational programmes

These are available to suit every taste. One of the most popular is that of the Higashi School, Boston: it is based on group activities led by the teacher and strictly structured and regimented exercises. It produces excellent results with regard to behaviour, but does not address problems in communication or social impairment. It is not a cure.

Rudolf Steiner schools suit some AS children, but have little effect on the key symptoms.

Home schooling, based on ABA therapy, may come close to a cure for most AS symptoms, but involves total commitment, including the time of the AS child's mother. It seems to have worked very well for Kenneth Hall, the author of *Asperger Syndrome, the Universe and Everything*, but he has the advantage of an exceptionally high IQ. Like other AS children, he prefers to learn for himself from books and his computer, or one-to-one, rather than in a group. He relates better to his laptop than to people.

Holding therapy

The theory behind this is that in autism there has been a fault or a stage missed out in the mother– baby bonding process. The aim is to reverse this by sessions of hugging the child so tightly that he struggles and rages. It is possible that this has the effect, like other forms of exercise, of releasing endorphins in the brain. These act like morphine, inducing a calm, contented feeling – temporarily. It has no effect on the basic symptoms of autism and has been criticized as a form of abuse.

The Squeeze Machine

Dr Temple Grandin is autistic and is an author and expert on the subject. She has invented the Squeeze Machine, based on the observation that cows produce more milk and cream if they are crammed together in their shed. Squeezing the feet is a simple way of using the machine. Closely wrapped bedclothes are an adjunct.

These two therapies provide the instinctive method of comforting, reassurance and the expression of love. The emotional aspects of AS are often mentioned, but rarely involved in treatment.

Complementary medicine

Alternative/complementary treatments are becoming more and more popular and accepted by traditional doctors. Most GPs refer some of their patients to alternative therapists, and a study was made by the OASIS organization of 45 alternative treatments; none was a cure for autism. No one can pinpoint how many of these therapies work, although there are numerous theories. The basic principle is to help both the body and mind to heal themselves.

Acupuncture

This is one of the most important complementary forms of treatment. It has been used since the Bronze Age of ancient China, and is applicable non-specifically to almost any condition that causes suffering, mental or physical.

Movement therapies

These are based on the theory that the body influences the mind as much as the other way round, and perhaps at a deeper level. The best-known techniques are *Rolfing*, founded by Ida Rolf; *Hellerwork* from Joseph Heller; and the most used one of all, *Feldenkrais*, worked out by a physicist, Mosche Feldenkrais. They all help with co-ordination, but have little other effects in AS.

Osteopathy and chiropractic

These have remained popular since the nineteenth century, both employing manipulation of the joints, with chiropractic involving the spine in particular. They provide some psychological as well as physical benefit.

Cranial osteopathy

This is now fashionable and credited by its adherents with having beneficial effects on autism.

The Alexander Technique

This is a method of moving and breathing that trains co-ordination and a sense of mental poise. It has been applied to almost everything including autism, and is a pleasant extra – but no more – in AS.

Naturopathy

Naturopathy is the essence of alternative medicine, using sun, air and water as therapy, but it works no miracles.

The Vision Theory

Paediatrician Mary Megson of the Autism Research Unit at Sunderland University believes that shortage of Vitamin A underlies symptoms of autism in some cases. Megson claims that this distorts the Asperger person's vision so that he cannot look other people in the eye. Language may also be affected. It is suggested that some children learn their words through the pictures on the television.

This can be corrected by taking cod liver oil, which contains Vitamin A, and the fish oils with the fatty acids omega 3 and 6. Paul Shattock, the director of the research unit, supports Ms Megson's theories, and although no scientific trials have been published, there have been striking individual cases of great improvement. However, the theory in general might seem too simplistic an explanation for something so diverse and complex as AS.

A boy of ten whose mother had night-blindness was thought to be autistic, and he had not spoken for six years. Because of his mother's problem, Ms Megson put the child on cod liver oil. After a few days he began taking notice of the pictures on the wall and running across the lawn where he would previously have kept carefully to the path. His sight was obviously improved, but more remarkably, after further administration of cod liver oil, he suddenly pointed to a jar of sweets and said: 'May I have a candy, please?' Language and sight both became normal. Shattock points out that shortage of cod liver oil cannot be the whole story, though, or no one in Norway (where they practically live on fish!) would ever have autism.

Encouraging special interests

There is a great deal we can all do to improve the lives of those with AS and other forms of autism, by building their self-confidence and enhancing their parents' pride and pleasure in their joint achievement – far more rewarding than hoping for miracles. For instance, encouraging and assisting an Aspie with his special interests has a sure-fire therapeutic effect. Popular subjects for AS people are computer science, TV, maths, space travel, timetables and electrical circuits.

Research has claimed that the beneficial effects of a special interest in children with AS run along the lines shown in Table 10.1.

Interest	80% (adults 64%)
Fun	73%
Security	65% (adults 32%)
Relaxation	62%
Reduced stress	55% (adults 38%)
More sociability	54%
Becoming an expert in the subject	32% (adults 36%)

Table 10.1.

The tilt test and swing therapy

The latest research from Florida, by O. and P. Teitelbaum, introduces two linked procedures. One is a quick and easy way to diagnose a potential for autism in very young children, and the other is a method of treatment. This is also quick and easy. Unbelievable? The Teitelbaums are well-established and well-respected researchers.

The tilt test

This is applicable from the age of six months onwards. The baby is held at an angle of 45 degrees, the tilt. Ordinary, neurotypical infants hold their heads vertically while their bodies are sloping, but those with the Asperger potential keep their heads in line with their bodies.

Swing therapy

This treatment consists of tilting the baby as in the test, then swinging him from side to side for ten minutes. This treatment is started as soon as there is a suspicion of autism. A daily session of swing therapy for two or three weeks is claimed to correct the tendency to autism.

It is difficult to see the connection between tilting, swinging and autism, but time and further trials may make this clearer. Meanwhile, we must go on applying the time-honoured treatments of love, patience and an open mind.

11

Lifestyle

Apart from the love, joy and laughter every little one brings with him, the impact of a child with AS on the family affects their whole lifestyle, down to the smallest detail. It is not a disaster, but can in fact be a benefit. It introduces structure and routine into what might otherwise be a confusing, chaotic set-up. The small boy – as we have seen, it is usually a boy – wants sameness and precision so passionately that the adults fall into line. Most of us grown-ups, even now, find that our familiar bedtime ritual relaxes us night after night. A routine helps the AS child in particular to feel safer, since they are always slightly anxious in a world where everyone else is operating on a different wavelength.

The structure of the day is held together by a skeleton of fixed points in a regular timetable of getting up, getting ready for school or playschool, breakfast, lunch and supper. Homework has its own slot as part of the home-from-school routine. This needs to involve a snack tea including some favourite item, and a short time to chat with Mother about the day before the homework stint.

Planning a routine

Most children like a break with routine, something new or different, like meeting new people, and visiting their homes. In contrast, AS children are more likely to throw a tantrum if such a 'treat' is sprung on them. The usual routine is not sacred, but any deviation calls for advance notice and planning. When Philip, featured in the case study below, was invited out to tea, his mother did not expect him to welcome the invitation, but realized that he would dread it as an ordeal. She made it easier by practising with him exactly what he should do and say, down to the exact wording of the final thanks.

It is important that the timing of regular events should not vary widely without forewarning. Planning is essential. It comes in two sizes: short-term and long-term.

Short-term planning covers what is to happen on the next day. It includes, for instance, what to eat. This can avoid a lot of argument at the table when the food is served. The youngster will have had his say at the planning stage, and if the menu includes something he cannot bear there must be an alternative, though not a special treat. AS children often have fads and idiosyncrasies that seem quite crazy about what they will or will not eat. Like girls with anorexia nervosa, they find the ordinary foods they do not want sickeningly revolting.

Christopher, the fictional AS hero of Mark Haddon's brilliant book *The Curious Incident of the Dog in the Night-time*, demonstrated a typical, incomprehensible refusal to eat if two different types of food were in contact on the plate or if they were yellow or brown.

Philip
Philip was seven. He would not touch anything orange or green, and it was sometimes difficult to accommodate these quirks. Philip's mother was worried lest he was not getting adequate nourishment. Planning was a help, but she had sometimes to resort to disguising one food with another. However, it is always risky not being as completely honest with an AS child as he is being with you.

Rituals and routines

Ian
Ian, aged eight, needed time to refocus after the stress of the social side of school. For him, the best way of doing this was to slip into a 15-minute routine of a drink of milk and three biscuits – one shortbread and two chocolate fingers – plus an exchange with his mum on the news of the day. This was followed by a session of homework and one TV programme. Bath-time and bedtime rituals rounded off Ian's day exactly the same as the day before.

Planning is made easier by establishing a precisely detailed routine or ritual – for instance, for getting up and dressing in the morning; having a bath; bedtime; and the home-from-school sequence. Play and TV come afterwards. The consequences game of 'When . . .' and 'Then . . .' is a useful ploy because it avoids giving direct commands which might invite resistance. Examples of this are: 'When you have eaten your egg, then you can have your ice cream' or 'When you've finished the maths, we'll go to the park and feed the ducks'.

Susie

Susie was 11, just entering puberty, when she developed a paralysing phobia of other people, especially if there were more than one or two of them. She panicked, with trembling and a thumping heart, when she had to meet a new person, and the problem became acute at the end of the school holidays when she had to face a different teacher and a different set of classmates. No one thought of AS as an underlying cause for the panics until it was noticed that comforting her did not help, nor telling her to 'tough it out'. Susie calmed down quickest if she was left alone, apart from inanimate objects like her computer, books and toys.

Tranquillizing medication made her feel better, but it has the disadvantage of being habit-forming. Planning ahead to avoid crowds and a half-hour wind-down time in her room after school were more effective.

Reminder cards

It helps youngsters to learn and practise routines if they list in writing the exact steps involved – for instance, a detailed plan of getting ready for school, what they need to take, such as dinner money or sandwiches, homework from the evening before, swimming gear, pens and pencils, etc. A particularly useful reminder spells out exactly what is meant by 'tidying your room' or behaving well in class.

Long-term planning

Something big, like a holiday, calls for careful preparation and discussion, so that the youngster knows what to expect and also what is expected of him. If the holiday involves being away from home, even for a day, this is the time for him to learn by heart (easy for an AS youngster) his name, address and phone number, and the words verbatim for approaching a lady or a policeman to ask for directions or other help.

Starting nursery school or big school is another project that requires advance planning and practice-runs at home. Mixing – and hopefully making friends – is an area that is particularly daunting for the AS youngster, but can be learned by rehearsal at home. It is more difficult for AS children to become accepted than for those with more severe types of ASD, who stand out as definitely odd. AS children are not obviously abnormal. They just don't fit in. Most of them are not interested in sport, especially football, and the subjects they are keen on are usually too adult to share with the general run of youngsters.

Pets

Pets are seldom mentioned in the many books and articles about bringing up children with AS, and developing the best in them. Yet they make a unique and valuable contribution to the happiness and well-being of the Aspie child. Or adult, come to that. Although he or she is likely to be confident and at ease with computers, DVDs, TV and mobiles, he is made anxious and unhappy by being misunderstood by people who are 'not on the same wavelength'.

Communing with a pet holds no such fears for the AS person. The dog or cat is smaller for a start, and has only a small repertoire of words he understands and a limited range of sounds he can make. People often do not understand what an animal is trying to convey, and you can see their frustration when they have been asking for food and some human being opens the back door for them instead.

Right away, the AS youngster is one step better off with the animal. Communicating with a pet, by stroking and patting on the one side and licking or purring on the other, is comforting and holds no threat. There is no risk of criticism or the small humiliations that bedevil exchanges with humans.

The most precious gifts from having a pet are the lessons in feelings. Emotional development is a vital part of growing up and learning responsibility for others who are weaker, practising loving care, and enjoying the sense of being loved in return. A dog or cat usually makes the best pet as it is already keen to get close to its humans, but any living creature can be rewarding and a comfort when the rest of the world does not understand. From pets, young humans learn about love, the top emotion, and its cousin, empathy.

There is a definite possibility that an AS child will develop a new routine: feeding, grooming and petting their animal and, in the case of gerbils, mice, hamsters and rabbits, cleaning out their cages. Let's hope so anyway.

A small extra bonus from playing with a pet is the pleasure of stroking its fur. As we have seen, the sense of touch is often unpleasantly acute in AS, but that does not seem to apply if it is an animal friend.

Plants

Growing plants that are edible, such as mustard-and-cress and radishes, brings children closer to nature. A delight in living things, plant or animal, does something to balance today's obsession with electronic equipment and the AS youngster's preference for communicating through it, to the detriment of his already impaired skill in this area.

Reading

This is an essential part of the lifestyle in a family with an AS member. Some AS children learn to read with hardly any help at a very early age. This is known as *hyperlexia*. Andrew, for example, could read the words of *The Times* at the age of three, but did not properly understand the politics underlying them. Today it is becoming commonplace for three-year-olds to learn to read and write with word-processors, but this has not ousted the convenience of reading from books – so portable, requiring no apparatus, and private. No one knows what you were reading when you close the book. AS youngsters appreciate this. They also like the extra information available on their special interests. Reading can also open the door of imagination.

While 99 per cent of Aspie children love reading, some of them have great difficulty in getting started. It is important to persist. Because of the way an Asperger brain works, it is not unusual for the whole penny to drop quite suddenly after months or even years of fruitless teaching and trying. At seven and a half, Luke Jackson was assessed as untestable – he could not read a word. A few days after this assessment, to his teacher's amazement, she discovered him reading a Shakespeare play fluently – by himself. And, as we have already seen, at 13 he wrote *Freaks, Geeks and Asperger Syndrome*.

Learning to read always involves mothers as well as teachers: no one else would have the patience to work with the youngster day after day, even when progress is at a snail's-pace. Sometimes the sessions need sweetening by munching a chocolate bar or, more healthily, an apple. Do not give up, however long it takes.

Reading aloud to each other (Mum and youngster) makes it more fun, and has the added benefit of developing clear articulation, and ironing out the common oddities in AS children's speech. These can be irritating to other people and sometimes incomprehensible, too soft or too loud, squeaky-high or a deadly, boring monotone.

Reading is best learned by AS children in complete words or phrases, and they do not have to be short and easy like 'cat and mat', as learned by many neurotypical children. The language of the Beatrix Potter books hits the right note for AS learners: short, simple, beautifully illustrated stories employing a scatter of long, adult words. AS children are often fascinated by these words and will pounce on each new one, as part of their collecting instinct.

They learn better and faster through their eyes than their ears, so it is good to have books with plenty of pictures. A hundred years ago even books for adults were illustrated – for instance, the Bible and all the novels by Dickens. Now we often have to make do with an occasional picture on the jacket. AS readers are likely to enjoy most books about science and mathematical puzzles and their own special subjects. Kenneth Hall, at ten, was keen to read books to learn about the still unsolved puzzle of pi. The exception to this is the fictional magic of Harry Potter's adventures, which works for all children, including those with AS.

Manners and communication

The words 'good manners' and 'politeness' may have a Victorian ring, but 'social communication' does not sound like a friendly way of dealing with other people. Good manners are the oil that helps people to get on with each other, especially in awkward situations.

For AS youngsters, manners are also a safeguard against accidentally offending others. However, your child may need to learn them by rote. It is handy to build up a bank of useful social phrases:

- Thank you for a lovely party, outing/game/present . . .
- What a delicious cake, ice cream, lunch, casserole . . .
- Congratulations on passing your exam.
- Are you better now? (after an illness)
- Would you like to play?

- May I join in?
- Excuse me – can you tell me the way to . . .

If you see someone in difficulty, or looking unhappy:

- Are you OK?
- Can I help you?
- Is it hurting you?

Other areas where your child may need guidance include:

- *Being 'a good sport'* – especially important at school. Explain to your child this means not sulking or moaning if he loses in a game, but remembering to say 'Well done' to the winner.
- *Table manners* – to stay at the table while other people are still eating, or to murmur 'Excuse me' when he gets down, to wait for everyone to be served before eating, or to pass the sugar or salt.
- *Letter writing* – a kind of 'polite conversation' is a formal letter of thanks for a present, sympathy for a loss, or congratulations for passing an exam. Explain that these can be very short, but are polite.
- *General good manners* – these include not crowding and pushing to get through a doorway, not taking someone else's place in a queue, and of course not saying or shouting rude words.
- *Managing anger* – encourage him or her to do something else that uses muscle power, like running round the garden or telling their difficulties to someone who will listen.

Making friends

One of the main benefits of mastering social skills is that it eases the route to making friends, something that does not come naturally to AS youngsters. Luke Jackson, author of *Freaks, Geeks and Asperger Syndrome*, has advice about this for other children. First he makes it clear that it is normal for an AS person, and perfectly acceptable, not to want a gang of friends, although most people want a few.

Hints on making friends:

- Look out for another loner.
- Don't be worried by a rebuff: the other guy would not have been much fun anyway!

- Learn to like yourself.
- Wear fashionable gear so long as you are comfortable in it.
- Make an effort to get on with anyone you are introduced to.

Rules for conversation could include:

- Don't stand too close to the other person: he needs space.
- Don't speak too loudly or too softly.
- Look at the person you are talking with.
- Be polite and don't say anything that might hurt his feelings (better to say nothing).
- Don't monopolize the conversation; remember to take turns in talking.
- Avoid going on for too long about your particular interest.

Asperger people are past masters at misinterpreting simple requests. 'Can you shut the window?' may be understood as 'Are you able to?' or 'Will you shut the window?' Or it may be taken as a criticism. It is better socially to combine any necessary criticism with asking for advice or mixing it with praise: 'Do you think we ought to turn the TV down a bit? You are so good at tuning it just right.'

Your child may also need advice on the delicate matter of compliments and telling the truth. Personal remarks can be a minefield. Admiring someone's appearance goes down well, as does praising their appearance, skill, tact or courage. Truthful but unflattering comments do not – for instance, about weight, laddered tights or undone buttons. 'Mind blindness' is an outlook AS children often have to grapple with. Home truths are just interesting to an AS person who cannot see how they may make the other party feel bad. You may need to explain that often being tactful means saying things that are not quite true in order not to hurt someone's feelings – the 'white lies' of the neurotypical world. For example, your child doesn't need to tell the world if he doesn't like Auntie's special home-made cake. Kindness is sometimes more important than accuracy.

12

Great thinkers with autistic characteristics

Isaac Newton, Albert Einstein and Bill Gates of Microsoft all had a difficult time as children because nobody understood them. With hindsight, it has been suggested that they each showed characteristics of Asperger Syndrome. What distinguishes AS people from others is their unusual way of thinking and of interpreting what goes on around them. The questions that bug an AS mind are deeper, more basic and of a different quality from those asked by most neurotypicals. Fundamental, sometimes previously unheard-of questions are raised – for instance, why the sky is blue or the final analysis of pi.

It is not surprising that in a group of children of high intelligence but with subtle or obvious anomalies of brain development a few may be exceptional – the geniuses. Others will have serious learning difficulties, but the majority will have an IQ moderately above average. Aptitude varies from one subject to another in the same person, and it is noticeable that brilliance in one area is often accompanied by deficiency in another – as in AS children with co-morbid conditions such as AD/HD or OCD.

There are two points to bear in mind:

1 Slow developers are by no means the same as 'being slow' or slow-witted.
2 Slow brain development is common in these exceptional people: 'the child who is backward today may be the genius of tomorrow'.

Famous people

Isaac Newton (1642–1727), arguably the greatest brain of all time, discovered, by pure thought, the rules of gravity governing our universe. His explanation was perfect – almost – but two centuries later Albert Einstein's theory of relativity filled in the gaps. Newton's early years were disappointing, and his ideas were dismissed as too far-fetched. He was consistently bottom of the class in Grantham Grammar School, mainly as a result of inattention: the

AD of AD/HD. His major work was his *Philosophae Naturalis Principia Mathematica.*

Other markedly slow developers include Einstein. When he was young he was seen as mentally slow, unsociable and a dreamer. Sometimes a child appears to be slow-witted when in fact he is taking extreme care in the accuracy of any answers he gives. Oliver Goldsmith, the eighteenth-century Irish playwright, novelist and poet, was assessed by his teachers as a 'stupid blockhead, whom everybody made fun of'.

Like many AS children, some of the slow starters had no interest in subjects in the school curriculum and would not waste time and effort unless they could see some point in them. Charles Darwin was one such. His father thought he was dull-witted and felt that the voyage on the *Beagle* would give him something to do that did not require great intelligence.

Other slow starters who did not find the subject they were to excel in early on included Manet, Marconi, Delius, Michael Faraday, Sir Henry Wood, Elgar, Gladstone, and Lord Northcliffe.

Particular difficulties

Mathematics are the stumbling block for many neurotypical children, but they are more likely to be a favourite subject for AS children. Exceptions were Schubert, Epstein, Conan Doyle, and Alfred Adler, while Gandhi never mastered his tables. Carl Jung could do calculations, but never stopped worrying about what the numbers really meant and whether they were facts. This is the kind of puzzle that typically preoccupies AS people. Rather similarly, Henri Poincaré, the renowned mathematician, had the curious defect of being unable to comprehend spatial relations, including geometry. He scored nil for drawing in his school entrance exam. He could not draw anything recognizable, even a square.

Problems with the development of language and speech are among the most frequent in children with AS, and also others with high intelligence. Stutterers are thought to include Moses, Aristotle, King Charles I, Aneurin Bevan and Michael Faraday. Somerset Maugham stammered all his life, and had a wretched time at school because of it.

Some AS and other children speak indistinctly because of imperfect development. Faraday pronounced 'r' as 'w' and Emile Zola pronounced his name 'Thola'. Neither Alessandro Volta, the Italian physicist, nor Einstein spoke at all until they were four, while

Wittgenstein, the philosopher, was nearly five. Einstein was still having difficulties at the age of seven, but reading and spelling caused many more problems for him than speech.

Dyslexia

A difficulty with reading and spelling is so common in AS that it is often regarded as symptomatic of the condition. John Hunter, the spoilt and youngest of three brothers, was regarded as 'impenetrable' to any form of book learning, a 'surly dullard, irredeemable by punishment or reward', and was assumed to be intellectually subnormal. He was put to work on a farm until he was 17 when he finally learned to read. He then assisted his anatomist brother, became fired with enthusiasm for medicine, and eventually became a distinguished surgeon. A similar passionate involvement in one subject is not unusual in AS youngsters.

The South African statesman Jan Smuts was 12 when he first learned to read, and George Stephenson, the famous railway engineer, never really grasped it. George Bernard Shaw always spelled phonetically; and Napoleon, Henry Ford, and Sir Joshua Reynolds were lifelong bad spellers. Despite the efforts of his aunts, Yeats experienced great difficulty in reading, and his father finally threw a book at his head.

Turner and Beethoven both had difficulty in expressing themselves in speech or writing, although they were brilliant in their own subjects. Some AS children have the same problem, together with difficulties in non-verbal communication. Poor communication is one of their basic triad of impairments.

Difficulties with languages, modern or classical, affected the Duke of Wellington; in fact, he had to leave Eton and do his military training in France. Linnaeus, surprisingly, was the worst in his school at Greek and Hebrew. Thomas Carlyle left university without a degree because of his weakness in classics, while Lord Lytton regarded Latin and Greek as 'inventions of some enemy of youthful happiness, involving special ordeals of torture like learning by heart'. Darwin said he had a lifelong inability to master any language, and Wagner was moved down a form because of his poor classics – and eventually stopped going to school. His parents did not know this until the teacher informed them that Richard had not attended school for six months!

Clumsiness

Most children and adults with AS show some impairment of muscle co-ordination – they are often dreadfully clumsy, awkward, or have a curious gait. Some brilliant men and women have had this developmental fault, an indication that AS was probably the underlying problem.

Napoleon could not throw a stone where he wanted, fire a gun accurately, or do his hair in the fashion of the times. Beethoven, Oscar Wilde and Trollope were always dropping and breaking things – and being teased for it. G. K. Chesterton's efforts at gymnastics were so odd that his friends gathered around to watch his antics. Fortunately, he took this in good part. Jung had similar problems with doing physical exercises.

Personal untidiness is inevitable where there is poor co-ordination, and this applies to Wilde and Trollope in particular, and also to those with AS. This is one reason for their lack of interest in their appearance – even among the teenage girls.

A similar developmental quirk is responsible for an abnormality that is a gift rather than a handicap: the ability to write or draw with either hand or both simultaneously. Leonardo da Vinci wrote fluently in mirror writing, from right to left. Baden Powell drew portraits of his friends using both hands, and Branwell Brontë could write Greek with his left hand and Latin with the right, at the same time. It is perhaps a pity that such enormous efforts are made to make clones of our children educationally. Parents of children with AS are especially privileged in having such unusual and interesting offspring. As we have already noted, Alessandro Volta, immortalized in the term 'voltage', was considered 'dull-witted' as a child, but his father admitted later: 'We had a jewel in our home but did not know it.' This is sometimes the situation with an AS child.

Tantrums and rages

Outbursts of anger are not uncommon in AS, and are often set off by unrecognized anxiety or frustration. Some famous men who may have had AS showed the same lack of control – for instance, Beethoven, Dean Inge, Goethe, Shelley, Cézanne and Wordsworth.

Those of us who are concerned with AS people know that their difficulty is not in loving and caring, but in expressing such feelings. Frustration and anxiety, which frequently plague AS youngsters, can lead to a loss of emotional control and tantrum-like behaviour, often with screaming, as it may in neurotypical children. There is sometimes misunderstanding of this, in that others may fear physical violence from AS youngsters. This is quite unjustified; in fact, usually an AS child is a victim, and likely to be criticized for being too timid and submissive.

Epilepsy

This brain disorder can affect babies and older people, including some with AS. Many great minds have had this handicap: Alexander the Great; our home-grown Alfred the Great: Pythagoras the mathematician; Julius Caesar; Napoleon; Van Gogh the artist; Pascal; and Paganini.

Just not 'fitting in'

Despite all the specific difficulties that occur in AS children in particular, the most typical is just 'not fitting in' as a result of the basic problem of not understanding other people's feelings, especially those of the peer group. This difficulty makes them seem arrogant and uncaring. Friedrich Nietzsche, the poet and philosopher, had qualities that may have been those of AS. He was, like most AS youngsters, 'serious, thoughtful and careful of his manners'. Other children made fun of his 'priggishness' and he did not have a single friend, in a strange, unsympathetic world. He had the literal, factual outlook that is a feature of AS. When a violent storm broke out when he was on his way home from school and all the other boys scuttled home like rabbits, Friedrich walked along sedately, covering his slate with his cap. His mother called out to him to hurry. When he got back she asked him why he did not run. He explained that the school rules forbade the boys from running about in the street, but said that they should walk home 'quickly and decorously'.

Nietzsche preferred solitude and 'the company of his own thoughts' to playing games. By the age of nine, he had written 55 poems. His mother was worried because he was different from other boys, but his grandfather said that he was a talented ugly duckling who might well turn out to be a swan!

The poet William B. Yeats was also a loner. He was shy and sensitive, easily rebuffed, and a sitting target for bullies. He was ashamed of being a coward. By the age of seven, he would have fitted a diagnosis of AS today, but in 1865 no one had heard of such a thing. It is sad to think of all these sensitive, talented children being classed as subnormal and misunderstood, and their parents worrying but not knowing what to do.

Particular 'brainboxes' who did not fit in

This group of brilliant men were notably awkward to get on with and failed in their personal and sentimental relationships, and in those with working colleagues.

Ludwig Josef Johann Wittgenstein

Ludwig Wittgenstein (1889–1951) was the eighth and youngest child of a Roman Catholic mother and father who had converted to Protestantism. The family was extremely wealthy and at the centre of Viennese culture: they had seven grand pianos! The children were educated at home until they were all 14. Ludwig was then sent to a non-academic school. He had been a very late talker and never learned to spell properly. He did not want friends or relationships and found the company of uncultured, working people almost physically painful. From 1908 to 1911 he studied engineering in Manchester, but became enthralled by the work of the mathematical philosopher, essayist and logician, Bertrand Russell. Russell delighted the thinkers, but upset the establishment with his pacifist and other unfashionable views. He lost his professorship over some pamphlets he had written on science, sex and war.

To study under Russell, Wittgenstein moved to Cambridge where he worked with 'passionate, profound, intense and domineering' interest. His focused mind and his preference for solitariness suggest he may have had AS. Russell came from a well-heeled aristocratic family but, like Wittgenstein, he was a slow developer, only emerging from adolescence and developing adult relationships in his thirties. For both these men, family riches and cultural connections facilitated their following the deeper levels of thought, like the Greeks of classical antiquity, who, similarly, did not have to struggle for a livelihood. In their case, the country was so fertile that no one had to work hard.

In 1913 Wittgenstein went to Norway to spend two years in solitude to think about logic. Then he joined the Austrian army to experience living 'eye to eye with death'. He also tried to catch typhoid for the same purpose. He felt he had no right to live unless he achieved some great work. His major work was his 70-page booklet: *Tractarius Logico-philosophicus*.

Twice he fancied himself to be in love, but neither time was this more than a peripheral thought. He felt it was of little importance compared with his fixation on the logical essence and philosophy of language. In typically AS mode, Wittgenstein dressed in a slovenly way and would only eat in the cheapest eating houses. He worked as a teacher by the curious method of thinking out loud about whatever came into his head: this was to ensure that the ideas were fresh and original. His lessons were not popular, nor was he. He had two friends, Keynes the economist and Ben Richards, a thinker who was 40 years his junior.

Anton Bruckner and Béla Bartók

At the turn of the nineteenth and twentieth centuries, two Hungarians, Anton Bruckner and Béla Bartók, each took a completely new line on musical composition, founding it on mathematical calculations, much as the computer 'nerds' of today apply their electronic obsession to the arts. As we have seen, OCD (see page 60) is often one aspect of AS.

Edmund Gosse

The poet Edmund Gosse (1845–1928) might have been labelled AS today. He never played with other children and claimed that he had not exchanged two words with anyone of his own age until he was eight years old. As often happens with AS children, he preferred the company of people who were much older or younger than he was. His parents were bigoted, God-fearing folk, and his father told Edmund that if he worshipped an idol made of wood or stone God would immediately manifest his anger. Taking things literally and curiosity are common traits in AS. Edmund tried saying his prayers to a chair, but nothing happened. Did he have AS or was he just eccentric?

Further reading

Attwood, Tony (1998) *Asperger's Syndrome: A Guide for Parents and Professionals.* London: Jessica Kingsley Publishers.

Bashe, Patricia Romanowski, and Kirby, Barbara L. (2001) *The OASIS Guide to Asperger Syndrome: Advice, Support, Insight and Inspiration.* New York: Crown Publishers.

Boyd, Brenda (2003) *Parenting a Child with Asperger Syndrome: 200 Tips and Strategies.* London: Jessica Kingsley Publishers.

Frith, U. (1991) *Autism and Asperger Syndrome.* Cambridge: Cambridge University Press.

Grandin, T. (1995) *Thinking in Pictures and Other Reports of my Life with Autism.* New York: Vintage Books.

Hall, K. (2000) *Asperger Syndrome, the Universe and Everything.* London: Jessica Kingsley Publishers.

Holliday Willey, L. (1999) *Pretending to be Normal: Living with Asperger Syndrome.* London: Jessica Kingsley Publishers.

Illingworth, R. S. and C. M. (1966) *Lessons from Childhood: Some Aspects of the Early Life of Unusual Men and Women.* Edinburgh: E. & S. Livingstone Publishers.

Jackson, Luke (2001) *A User Guide to the GF/CF Diet for Autism, Asperger Syndrome and AD/HD.* London: Jessica Kingsley Publishers.

Jackson, Luke (2003) *Freaks, Geeks and Asperger Syndrome: A User Guide to Adolescence.* London: Jessica Kingsley Publishers.

Moore, Charlotte (2004) *George and Sam: Autism in the Family.* London: Viking.

Seroussi, K. (2000) *Unravelling the Mystery of Autism ad Pervasive Developmental Disorder: A Mother's Story of Research and Recovery.* New York: Simon & Schuster.

Smith Myles, Brenda, and Adreon, Diana (2001) *Asperger Syndrome and Adolescence: Practical Solutions for School Success.* New York: Autism Asperger Publishing.

Useful addresses

Allergy induced Autism (A i A)

11 Larklands
Longthorpe
Peterborough PE3 6II
UK
Tel: 01733 331771

Asperger Syndrome Coalition of the US

ASC-US, Inc.
PO Box 49267
Jacksonville Beach
FL 32240
USA
Tel: 866 4ASPRGR or 866 427 7747

Asperger's Syndrome Support Network

C/o VACCA
PO Box 235
Ashburton
Victoria 3147
Australia

Autism Research Unit

School of Sciences (Health)
University of Sunderland
Sunderland SR2 7EE
UK
Tel: 0191 510 8922

Autism Society of America

7910 Woodmont Avenue
Suite 300
Bethesda
MD20814–3015
USA
Tel: 800 3AUTISM or 301 657 0881

Autism Society of Canada

129 Yorkville Avenue, Suite 202
Toronto
Ontario MR5 1C4
Canada
Tel: 416 922 0302

Autistic Association of New Zealand

c/o Box 7305
Sydenham
Christchurch
New Zealand
Tel: 03 332 1038

Home Education Advisory Service (HEAS)

PO Box 98
Welwyn Garden City
Herts AL8 6AN
UK
Tel: 01707 371654

Hyperactive Children Support Group (HACSG)

71 Whyke Lane
Chichester
West Sussex PO19 2LD
UK
Tel: 01903 725182

National Association for Gifted Children

540 Elder House
Milton Keynes MK9 1LR
UK
Tel: 01908 673677

National Autistic Society

393 City Road
London EC1V 1NG
UK
Tel: 020 7833 2299

Parents and Professionals and Autism
(The Northern Ireland Autism Charity)
Knockbracken Healthcare Park
Saintfield Road
Belfast BT8 8BH
Northern Ireland

Websites

Autism Research Centre
www.psychiatry.cam.uk

Bullying Online
www.bullying.co.uk

Dyspraxia Foundation
www.dyspraxiafoundation.org.uk/

Home Education Link for the UK
www.he-special.org.uk

Hyperlexia
www.hyperlexia.org

National Attention Deficit Disorder Association
www.add.org/

National Autistic Society
www.oneworld.org/autism_uk/index.html

OASIS (Online Asperger Syndrome Information and Support)
www.udel.edu/bkirby/asperger/

Obsessive Compulsive Disorder Foundation
www.ocfoundation.org/

Tony Attwood
www.tonyattwood.com

University Students with Autism and Asperger's Syndrome
www.cns.dicon.co.uk

World Taekwondo Federation
www.kukkiwon.or.kr

Resources for home education in the UK

Choice in Education

Group promoting home schooling. Runs the Home Educators' Seaside Festival (camping, workshops, discussions, games). Newsletters.
PO Box 20284, London NW1 3WY
Website: www.choiceineducation.co.uk

Education Otherwise (EO)

Support for home-educators seeking for the best match for individual children's needs and parents' beliefs. SAE to:
PO Box 7420, London N9 9SG
Website: www.education-otherwise.org

Free Range Education

Practical advice, including legal, about home education, local groups, reading list, etc.
Website: www.free-range-education.co.uk

HE-special-UK e-mail list

A supportive meeting place for families home-educating their children.
Website: www.he-special.org.uk

Herald

Offers a flexible framework as a basis for study. For details write to:
Herald, Kelda Cottage, Lydbrook, Glos GL17 9SX
Tel: 01594 861107
Website: www.homeeducation.co.uk

Home Education Advisory Service (HEAS)

Support and advice to parents wishing to home-educate their children. Publishers of *The Big Book of Resource Ideas* and *The Home Education Handbook*. Subscribers receive a quarterly bulletin.
HEAS PO Box 98, Welwyn Garden City, Herts AL8 6AN
Tel/Fax: 01707 371 854
E-mail: enquiries@heas.org.uk
Website: www.heas.org.uk

Independent Panel for Special Education Advice

Advice line: 0800 0184016
General enquiries: 01394 380518

Schoolhouse

Scottish charity giving support and information to home-educators.
Enquiry line, newsletter, young people's newspaper, teenage support
network. Voluntary donation for membership.
Schoolhouse Home Education Association,
311 Perth Road, Dundee DD2 1LG
Tel: 0870 1968; information: 0870 1967
E-mail: info@schoolhouse.org.uk
Website: www.schoolhouse.org.uk

Spearhead

An independent charity giving free advice and support to parents
considering home-schooling.
Tel: 0161 7244
E-mail: advice.spearhead@lineone.net

Appendix: Criteria for a definitive diagnosis of Asperger Syndrome

1 Difficulty in relating to other people, or 'impaired social interaction'. This is demonstrated by at least two of the following:

- Poor non-verbal communication, which means facial expressions such as smiling, laughing, frowning, crying or grimacing, and other meaningful movements, postures or gestures. Clenching the fists, stamping or kicking are threats, while shaking hands, kissing and hugging convey affection. Clapping means 'well done'.
- Does not mix easily or make friends with others of the same age.
- Makes no effort to share his interests, pleasures or work projects.
- Does not respond to approaches by others, as in conversation.

2 Limited range of stereotyped and repetitive actions and interests, as shown by at least one of the following:

- Preoccupation of great intensity with one or a few special interests: he may not talk about anything else at all.
- Inflexible routines and rituals that appear to serve no useful purpose and cause anxiety or anger if they are interrupted.
- Motor mannerisms involving fingers, hands or the whole body.
- Fascination with parts of objects.

3 The symptoms interfere with social, family, and school or work life.
4 No significant delay in the development of thinking and logic, including curiosity about his environment and the acquisition of the skills of everyday living.
5 No general delay in language development. For instance, the child can say single words by the age of two, and two- or three-word phrases for communication when he is three.
6 The criteria do not fit any other specific developmental disorder or schizophrenia.

Autistic Spectrum Disorder, ASD, of which Asperger Syndrome, AS, is a member, is becoming increasingly frequent – and important.

It is now more common than childhood cancer, Down's syndrome, muscular dystrophy or cerebral palsy, affecting 1 in 250–500 children. It can be just as crippling in a different way.

Index